Dispelling the Myths About Addiction

Strategies to Increase Understanding and Strengthen Research

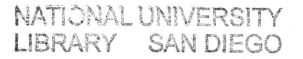

Committee to Identify Strategies to Raise the Profile of
Substance Abuse and Alcoholism Research

Division of Neuroscience and Behavioral Health

Division of Health Promotion and Disease Prevention

INSTITUTE OF MEDICINE

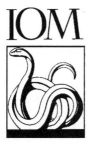

NATIONAL ACADEMY PRESS
Washington, D.C. 1997

NATIONAL ACADEMY PRESS • 2101 Constitution Avenue, N.W. • Washington, DC 20418

NOTICE: The project that is the subject of this report was approved by the Governing Board of the National Research Council, whose members are drawn from the councils of the National Academy of Sciences, the National Academy of Engineering, and the Institute of Medicine. The members of the committee responsible for the report were chosen for their special competences and with regard for appropriate balance.

This report has been reviewed by a group other than the authors according to procedures approved by a Report Review Committee consisting of members of the National Academy of Sciences, the National Academy of Engineering, and the Institute of Medicine.

The Institute of Medicine was chartered in 1970 by the National Academy of Sciences to enlist distinguished members of the appropriate professions in the examination of policy matters pertaining to the health of the public. In this, the Institute acts under both the Academy's 1863 congressional charter responsibility to be an adviser to the federal government and its own initiative in identifying issues of medical care, research, and education. Dr. Kenneth I. Shine is president of the Institute of Medicine.

This study was supported under a grant from the W.M. Keck Foundation of Los Angeles. The views presented are those of the Institute of Medicine Committee to Identify Strategies to Raise the Profile of Substance Abuse and Alcoholism Research and are not necessarily those of the funding organization.

Library of Congress Catalog Card No. 97-69691
International Standard Book Number 0-309-06401-5

Additional copies of this report are available from:

National Academy Press
2101 Constitution Avenue, N.W.
Lock Box 285
Washington, DC 20055

Call 800-624-6242 or 202-334-3313 (in the Washington metropolitan area) or visit the National Academy Press's online bookstore at **http://www.nap.edu**.

The serpent has been a symbol of long life, healing, and knowledge among almost all cultures and religions since the beginning of recorded history. The image adopted as a logotype by the Institute of Medicine is based on a relief carving from ancient Greece, now held by the Staatlichemuseen in Berlin.

Cover: The cover of this report includes a circular motif, called a mandala, that was designed by Leigh Coriale of the National Academy Press. The term *mandala* comes from Sanskrit, and such motifs are prominent among many of the world's religions. In psychology, mandalas were studied and used most extensively by the psychiatrist Carl Jung, who viewed mandalas as abstract representations of the totality of the conscious and unconscious. Universal elements of the unconscious, or archetypes, were important in Jung's theory of individual psychological development and manifestations, but also were evident in symbols, myths, legends, and rituals. Color reprints of some of Jung's patient's madalas are contained in R.F.C. Hull's English translation of Jung's book, *The Archetypes and the Collective Unconscious* (Second Edition, Tenth Printing; Princeton, NJ: Princeton University Press, 1990).

STEPHEN M. WEISS, Professor and Codirector, Division of Behavioral Medicine and Consultation Psychiatry, School of Medicine, University of Miami, Miami, Florida

Institute of Medicine Staff

LAUREN B. LEVETON, Study Director until September 1996
CARRIE E. INGALLS, Research Associate
THOMAS J. WETTERHAN, Project Assistant/Research Assistant
AMELIA B. MATHIS, Project Assistant
TERRI SCANLAN, Administrative Assistant
DIANA ZUCKERMAN, Consultant
MICHAEL A. STOTO, Director, Division of Health Promotion and Disease Prevention
CONSTANCE M. PECHURA, Director, Division of Neuroscience and Behavioral Health

Preface

Research on addiction reveals fascinating paradoxes and contradictions. On one hand, there are enormous opportunities, such as those for furthering knowledge about the complex and sophisticated science of neurobiology. Scientists have identified many of the brain mechanisms that lead human beings to develop the cravings and physical dependencies that characterize addiction. These mechanisms appear to be at work with many different types of drugs, ranging from commonly used legal drugs, such as nicotine, to illicit drugs, such as heroin, which are abused and, in some individuals, lead to addiction.

There are enormous barriers, however, based on stigma and misunderstanding, which have undermined the benefits of increased scientific knowledge. To address this problem effectively, the public, health educators, policymakers, and clinicians who treat addiction must be educated about research accomplishments and critical questions, and additional researchers must be recruited into the field. This report attempts to identify key barriers that need to be overcome before a rational, science-based approach to drug addiction, one of our most pressing public health problems, can be achieved.

Many Institute of Medicine (IOM) studies are intended to serve as instruments of change that will shape future policies. The charge to the Committee on Raising the Profile of Substance Abuse and Alcoholism Research was to conduct a study and to develop a report to identify and address barriers to public understanding of the field and those that present obstacles for attracting and sustaining talented investigators and other health professionals who wish to pursue careers in addiction research. The committee was also charged with developing strategies to overcome the barriers.

As work on this study progressed, a novel situation unfolded: the process itself became a catalyst for change. Committee members learned from one another—basic researchers from clinical and behavioral researchers, senior from younger, and those outside the field from those within. In particular, a workshop held in March of 1996 brought committee members, young* and senior investigators, and other health professionals and policymakers together in a meeting that helped to begin changes in attitudes and increases in knowledge (see Appendix A for the workshop agenda and Appendix B for a list of participants). The workshop provided new insights, encouraged constructive debate, and ultimately achieved consensus about the various barriers; it also stimulated innovative thinking about critical strategies. The results of the workshop and committee deliberations are presented in this report, which we hope will also be an instrument of change. It is addressed to several audiences, but particularly to the lay public, college and graduate students, university administrators, policymakers, and others who may be interested in understanding drug abuse and addiction.

This report sets forth a strategy to dispel the myths about addiction and to facilitate a better understanding of the accomplishments in addiction research and the critical questions that remain to be answered (Chapters 3, 4 and 5). Addiction to nicotine, alcohol, and illegal drugs is a preventable and treatable brain disease influenced by complex sets of behaviors that may be the results of genetic, biological, psychosocial, and environmental interactions, as this report emphasizes. The costs of these problems are high and underscore the need to approach the problems from a perspective that is more rational and evidence based.

The committee of 16 members was carefully selected to represent basic, clinical, and behavioral researchers both inside and outside the field of drug addiction with expertise spanning different disciplines (e.g., neuroscience, psychopharmacology, anesthesiology, behavioral medicine, economics) and different substances (e.g., nicotine, alcohol, opioids, stimulants). They were also selected for their experience in careers associated with academia, government, and industry. In addition, to improve understanding as to how various barriers may pose problems at different stages of a research career, the committee was selected to be representative of those different stages, ranging from junior to more senior researchers and clinicians.

The committee collected quantitative and qualitative data during the study, including data on prevalence and costs of addiction (Chapter 2), efforts made in educational settings from early grades through medical schools (Chapter 6), investments in research and training (Chapter 7), and initiatives to educate the

---

*Young investigators were defined for the purpose of this study *not* by chronological age, but rather as individuals who were at early stages of their careers.

public and the role of public perception in supporting or inhibiting increased understanding and implementation of effective public policies regarding research (Chapter 8).

The day-and-a-half workshop was a major data gathering activity that helped to shape the search for information and enriched the committee discussions. The workshop highlighted young investigators' perceptions of their experiences of the barriers and opportunities in pursuing careers in addiction research and treatment. The young investigators represented the entire spectrum of career pathways, from predoctoral and premedical students to recent postdoctoral and junior faculty individuals. In addition, they represented career paths spanning neurobiological, clinical, and behavioral areas both inside and outside addiction research and treatment. The workshop also included a broad representation of other individuals—senior investigators inside and outside addiction research, and medical and health professionals and policymakers representing universities, foundations, industry, government, and professional associations interested in addiction research.

Seventy people participated in the workshop and an additional 29 young investigators and 25 senior investigators and other professionals provided written contributions about their perceptions and experiences of barriers and strategies for attracting individuals into the field (Appendix B contains the list of workshop participants and contributors). The committee also heard about advances in addiction research from two keynote speakers, Drs. Avram Goldstein and Ivan Diamond, who shared valuable perspectives based on their extensive experience in this field (Appendixes C and D). Finally, to obtain a perspective on lessons learned, three speakers described how their fields had advanced and overcome the barriers posed by stigma. The fields (depression, epilepsy, and breast cancer) were selected by the committee to illustrate success stories that could serve as role models for advancing the field of addiction research.

Many individuals helped the committee do its work, but first we would like to thank the W.M. Keck Foundation of Los Angeles for their financial support, without which this study would not have taken place. We would like to thank the committee members for their dedication and diligence, but most of all for their open-mindedness and flexibility. Each made a unique contribution and broadened our perspective. We also appreciate the efforts of a number of people who obtained and provided information on the various federal agencies and their funding, and shared their knowledge and perspectives through interviews and questionnaires. Several people provided valuable assistance in preparing chapter drafts, workshop summaries, and in copy editing the manuscript (Diana Zuckerman, Sara Brookhart, Peter Slavin, and Beth Gyorgy). Most particularly, we are grateful to the IOM staff: Lauren Leveton for assuming in-house leadership for the study and the organization of the workshop until September 1996; Constance Pechura for providing wise oversight; Carrie Ingalls for exceptional research and writing assistance; Thomas Wetterhan for additional skilled research support, manuscript preparation, and logistical support; Terri Scanlan for consistently helpful administrative assistance; and Amelia Mathis for making our travel, meeting arrangements and meals comfortable and enjoyable. Also, we appreciate the efforts of Michael Edington, managing editor, Claudia Carl, administrative associate for report review, and Carlos Gabriel, financial associate. Finally, we would like to thank all the young investigators who have much to look forward to as they pursue the exciting challenges in addiction research.

Nancy C. Andreasen M.D., Ph.D., *Chair*
Stanley Watson, M.D., Ph.D., *Vice-Chair*

Contents

SUMMARY   1

1 INTRODUCTION   11
Definitions and Concepts, 13
Classification of Drugs, 14
Organization of the Report, 16

2 PREVALENCE, COSTS, AND INVESTMENTS   19
Prevalence, 19
Economic Costs of Addiction, 25
Investments, 28
Conclusion, 32

3 NEUROBIOLOGY OF ADDICTION: AN OVERVIEW   37
The Brain's Common "Reward" Pathway, 39
Drug Effects on Brain Reward Systems, 41
Emotion, Memory, and the Transition from Use to Addiction, 42
Vulnerabilities to Addiction, 47
Conclusion, 49

4 PSYCHOSOCIAL FACTORS AND PREVENTION   55
Psychosocial Factors, 55
Prevention, 57
Conclusion, 66

5   TREATING ADDICTIVE DISORDERS   73
Treatments for Alcohol and Cocaine Addiction, 75
Treatments for Opioid Addiction, 83
Smoking Cessation Programs, 85
Conclusion, 87

6   EDUCATION AND TRAINING   95
Career Pathways, 96
Secondary School and Undergraduate Education, 97
Graduate and Professional Education, 99
The Importance of Mentors, 106
Specialization and Credentialing Issues, 109
Conclusion, 111

7   RESOURCES NEEDED FOR YOUNG INVESTIGATORS   115
Funding Levels, 119
The Pipeline, 120

8   PUBLIC PERCEPTIONS, PUBLIC POLICIES   139
Stigma, 139
Advocacy, 141
A Model for Understanding the Educational and Public Barriers, 142
Strategies, 142

APPENDIXES
A   Workshop Agenda, 149
B   Workshop Contributors and Participants, 153
C   Plenary Lecture I, *Avram Goldstein, M.D.*, 161
D   Plenary Lecture II, *Ivan Diamond, M.D., Ph.D.*, 169
E   History of Drug Addiction Research: Key Discoveries/Events, National
      Policies, and Funding, 177
F   Recent Advances in Addiction Research, 193
G   Recent Advances in Pharmacotherapy, 199
H   Recent Advances in Behavioral Sciences and Treatment, 201
I   Key Barriers and Critical Strategies in the Research and Public
      Arenas, 205

INDEX   211

TABLES, FIGURES, AND BOXES

Tables

1.1 Classification of Abusive and Addictive Drugs, 17
2.1 Trends in Past Month Use of Marijuana, Alcohol, and Cigarettes by 8th Graders, 10th Graders, and High School Seniors, 1992–1996, 24
2.2 Estimated Economic Costs of Illicit Drug, Alcohol, and Nicotine Abuse, 1990 (millions of dollars), 26
2.3 Costs of Illness for Selected Diseases and Conditions (billions of dollars), 29
2.4 NIDA Funding History (1988–1997): Research Training Grants, Research Grants, and Total Budget (thousands of dollars), 31
2.5 NIAAA Funding History (1988–1997): Research Training Grants, Research Grants, and Total Budget (thousands of dollars), 31
3.1 Some Future Challenges in Basic Research, 50
4.1 Some Future Challenges in Psychosocial and Prevention Research, 67
5.1 Duration of Addiction Treatment, 76
5.2 Some Future Challenges in Pharmacotherapy and Treatment Research, 88
7.1 Total Costs to Society and Training and Research Support for Specific Diseases (millions of dollars), 119
7.2 R01 Success Rates, 129
7.3 NIDA Research Training Funding as a Percentage of Total Extramural Research Funding (millions of dollars), 130
7.4 NIAAA Research Training Funding as a Percentage of Total Extramural Research Funding (millions of dollars), 130

Figures

2.1 Past month illicit drug use by age: 1979–1995, 20
2.2 Past month illicit drug use, by past month alcohol use, age 12 and older, 1995, 22
2.3 Economic costs of addiction by type of cost and drug, 1990, 27
3.1 Schematic diagram of the brain reward circuitry, 40
3.2 The effect of cocaine and amphetamine, 42
7.1 Total institute budgets, 1986–1995 (constant dollars), 122
7.2 Total institute research grant budgets, 1986–1995 (constant dollars), 123
7.3 Total research training grant budgets, 1986–1995 (constant dollars), 124
7.4 Total number of T32, F31, and F32 applicants, 1986–1995, 125
7.5 Total number of T32, F31, and F32 awards granted, 1986–1995, 126
7.6 Total number of R01 and R29 applicants, 1986–1995, 127
7.7 Total number of R01 and R29 awards granted, 1986–1995, 128

8.1 Critical links in the strategies for raising the profile of addiction research, 143

Boxes

2.1 Estimating the Cost of Drug Abuse in New York City, 28
3.1 Animal Models: Examples from Alcohol Research, 38
3.2 Effects of Alcohol on Neurotransmission, 43
6.1 American Association for the Advancement of Science, 98
6.2 Faculty for Undergraduate Neuroscience, 99
6.3 Case Study: Harvard Medical School, Division on Addictions, 102
6.4 Case Study: University of Pennsylvania, School of Medicine, 103
6.5 North Carolina Governor's Institute on Alcohol and Substance Abuse, Inc., 105
7.1 Description of Awards, 116
7.2 Foundation-Funded Research: A Model Program, 132

Acronyms

AA	Alcoholics Anonymous
AAAS	American Association for the Advancement of Science
AAMC	Association of American Medical Colleges
ABPN	American Board of Psychiatry and Neurology
ACS	American Cancer Society
ADA	American Diabetes Association
ADD	attention-deficit disorder
ADH	alcohol dehydrogenase
ADHD	attention-deficit hyperactivity disorder
AHA	American Heart Association
AHCPR	Agency for Health Care Policy and Research, United States Department of Health and Human Services
AHEC	Area Health Education Centers
AIDS	acquired immunodeficiency syndrome
ALDH2	aldehyde dehydrogenase
AMA	American Medical Association
AMERSA	Association for Medical Education and Research in Substance Abuse
APA	American Psychological Association
ASA	American Sociological Association
ASAM	American Society of Addiction Medicine
ATP	adenosine triphosphate
AVP	arginine vasopressin
B/START	Behavioral Science Track Award for Rapid Transition

BAC	blood alcohol concentrations
BLS	Bureau of Labor Statistics
cAMP	cyclic adenosine monophosphate
CASA	Center on Addiction and Substance Abuse
CCK-8	cholecystokinin-8
cDNA	deoxyribonucleic acid, complementary sequence
cm	centimeters
CME	continuing medical education
CNS	central nervous system
CRA	community reinforcement approach
CRF	corticotropin releasing factor
CSAP	Center for Substance Abuse Prevention
CSAT	Center for Substance Abuse Treatment
DARP	Drug Abuse Reporting Project
DEA	Drug Enforcement Administration
delta-9-THC	delta-9-tetrahydrocannabinol
DHHS	Department of Health and Human Services
DMT	dimethyltryptamine
DNA	deoxyribonucleic acid
DoD	Department of Defense
DOM	dimethoxymethylamphetamine
DOT	Department of Transportation
DSM-III-R	*Diagnostic and Statistical Manual of Mental Disorders—* Third Edition Revised
DSM-IV	*Diagnostic and Statistical Manual of Mental Disorders—* Fourth Edition
DWI	driving while intoxicated
F30	Individual Predoctoral National Research Service Award for M.D./Ph.D. Fellowships
F31	Individual Predoctoral National Research Service Award for Fellows
F32	Individual Postdoctoral National Research Service Award for Fellows
FAS	fetal alcohol syndrome
FDA	Food and Drug Administration
FHN	familial high-alcohol nonpreferring
FHP	familial high-alcohol preferring
FUN	Faculty for Undergraduate Neuroscience
GABA	gamma-aminobutyric acid
GAO	General Accounting Office
HCFA	Health Care Financing Administration
HCl	hydrochloride

HDL	high-density lipoprotein
HIV	human immunodeficiency virus
HRSA	Health Research and Services Administration
ICD	International Classification of Disease
IOM	Institute of Medicine
IRB	institutional review board
IRG	initial review group
K01	Mentored Research Scientist Development Award
K02	Independent Scientist Award
K05	Senior Scientist Award
K07	Academic Career Award
K08	Mentored Clinical Scientist Development Award
kcal	kilocalories
LAAM	levo-alpha-acetylmethadol or levomethadyl acetate, trade name: Orlaam®
LCME	Liaison Committee on Medical Education
LRP	Loan Repayment Program
LSD	lysergic acid diethylamide
LTA	latent transition analysis
MATCH	Matching Alcohol Treatment to Client Heterogeneity
MDA	methylenedioxyamphetamine
MDD	Medications Development Division
MDMA	methylenedioxymethamphetamine
mg	milligram
mm	millimeter
MMWR	*Morbidity and Mortality Weekly Report*
MOU	memorandum of understanding
MSTP	Medical Sciences Training Program
NAc	nucleus accumbens
NAMA	National Alliance of Methadone Advocates
NAMI	National Alliance for the Mentally Ill
NARSAD	National Alliance for Research on Schizophrenia and Depression
NAS	National Academy of Sciences
NBCC	National Breast Cancer Coalition
NCHGR	National Center for Human Genome Research
NCHS	National Center for Health Statistics
NCI	National Cancer Institute
NCRR	National Center for Research Resources
NEI	National Eye Institute
NHLBI	National Heart, Lung, and Blood Institute
NIA	National Institute on Aging

NIAAA	National Institute on Alcohol Abuse and Alcoholism
NIAID	National Institute of Allergy and Infectious Diseases
NIAMS	National Institute of Arthritis and Musculoskeletal and Skin Diseases
NICHD	National Institute of Child Health and Human Development
NIDA	National Institute on Drug Abuse
NIDCD	National Institute on Deafness and Other Communication Disorders
NIDDK	National Institute of Diabetes and Digestive and Kidney Diseases
NIDR	National Institute of Dental Research
NIEHS	National Institute of Environmental Health Sciences
NIGMS	National Institute of General Medical Sciences
NIH	National Institutes of Health
NIMH	National Institute of Mental Health
NINDS	National Institute of Neurological Disorders and Stroke
NINR	National Institute of Nursing Research
NMDA	N-methyl-D-aspartate
NRC	National Research Council
NRSA	National Research Service Awards
OER	Office of Extramural Research
ONDCP	Office of National Drug Control Policy
OTA	Office of Technology Assessment
OTC	over-the-counter
PCP	phencyclidine
PET	positron-emission tomography
PTSD	posttraumatic stress disorder
QTL	quantitative trait loci
R01	Investigator Initiated Research Project
R03	Small Grant
R21	Exploratory/Developmental Grant
R29	FIRST Award—First Independent Research Support and Transition Award
R37	MERIT Award—Method to Extend Research in Time Award
RFA	request for applications
RFP	request for proposals
RI	recombinant inbred
RWJF	Robert Wood Johnson Foundation
SAMHSA	Substance Abuse and Mental Health Services Administration
SOAR	The Society of American Recovery
SPECT	single photon emission computed tomography

T32	National Research Service Award Institutional Research Training Grant
T35	National Research Service Award Short-Term Institutional Research Training Grant
THC	tetrahydrocannabinol
TOPS	Treatment Outcomes Prospective Study
VTA	ventral tegmental area
WHO	World Health Organization

Summary

Addiction is a major public health problem. Although great strides have been made in understanding the nature of addiction and its genetic, biological, psychological, and environmental factors, addiction is not well understood by the public or by policymakers, and addiction research is often an undervalued and stigmatized area of inquiry. Overcoming these problems of stigma and misunderstanding will require educating the public, health educators, policymakers, and clinicians, highlighting progress made, and recruiting talented researchers into the field.

Multiple definitions and confusing terminology constitute one barrier that promotes misunderstanding about addiction and the need for research. This and other Institute of Medicine committees have defined drug addiction as a **brain disease** similar to other chronic, relapsing conditions, such as heart disease and diabetes, and manifested by a complex set of behaviors that are the result of genetic, biological, psychosocial, and environmental interactions.[1] The term "addiction" has tended to be applied more frequently to use of illegal drugs than to legal ones; yet, addiction may occur as a consequence of using both socially acceptable, legal drugs or illicit drugs. Four major classes of drugs (nicotine, alcohol, opioids, and stimulants) are emphasized because they have the greatest economic impact on society and cause, or contribute to, many life-threatening disorders, including heart disease, cirrhosis, AIDS, and cancer.[2]

PREVALENCE, COSTS, AND RESEARCH INVESTMENTS

Drug abuse has been called the nation's number one public health problem. Of the nation's personal health care expenditures, $1 of every $12 is spent on prevention, diagnosis, and treatment of people suffering from addictive diseases. The measurable total economic costs of drug addiction clearly are enormous, totaling $256.8 billion in 1990. Alcohol use, abuse, and addiction, including the direct costs of crime, motor vehicle crashes, and other related costs, comes at the highest cost, estimated at $98.6 billion. The cost of nicotine addiction follows ($91.3 billion), and then addiction to illegal drugs ($66.9 billion).

NEUROBIOLOGY OF ADDICTION: AN OVERVIEW

Recent discoveries have turned addiction research into a field that should attract the very best scientists interested in both basic and translational research. Researchers have cloned the brain receptors (i.e., the immediate molecular targets) for all significant drugs of abuse and have defined their locations in the brain. Of great significance, there is now general agreement on the importance of the dopaminergic brain reward pathway as one of the key common sites of action of addictive drugs. Some aspects of treatment for all drugs are beginning to capitalize on the identification of this common pathway and the systems that regulate it. Researchers can now turn to the very difficult problems of understanding the precise brain mechanisms by which drugs alter brain function and come to dominate behavior. In the process, a great deal will be learned about the normal control of motivation and emotion in the brain. With such discoveries, understandings about other human diseases and illnesses can also be gained. For example, dopamine systems are not only the substrates of drug abuse and addiction, but are also involved in a variety of psychiatric disorders and some movement disorders, such as Parkinson's disease.

The importance of these findings notwithstanding, it must be emphasized that drug addiction is the result of interacting biological, behavioral, social, and environmental factors. Thus, the development of successful treatments can come only from integrative, multidisciplinary research that may provide stronger connections between research and clinical practice.

PSYCHOSOCIAL FACTORS AND PREVENTION

How does the use of tobacco, alcohol, opioids, and stimulants begin? Virtually all Americans, some of whom may have a genetic vulnerability to drug abuse, are faced with the decision of whether to smoke, drink alcohol, or take illicit drugs. Why do some individuals say yes and others refuse? In addition to studies about genetic vulnerabilities, these and similar questions are the focus of behavioral, epidemiological, and social science research aimed at understanding and preventing drug addiction. Psychosocial factors include personality, as well as family, peer, and other environmental factors that either increase the risk of an individual developing an addictive disorder (risk factors) or decrease such risks (protective factors). Research indicates that beliefs and attitudes, many of which are learned by watching or listening to role models at home, in the community, or in the media, have a strong influence on drug use and abuse. As a result, changing the environmental conditions or cues associated with drug use or withdrawal can assist an individual's efforts to abstain from drugs.

By using cognitive and behavioral research regarding the psychosocial factors related to drug initiation and use, prevention interventions have been and continue to be developed. Prevention interventions can be *universal, selective,* or *indicated* as defined by a previous Institute of Medicine (IOM) committee. Universal includes interventions aimed toward an entire population, such as warning labels on tobacco products and alcoholic beverages, advertising bans, smoke-free airline flights and buildings, taxes, and the role of primary care physicians and providers in inquiring about and providing information on smoking, drinking, and use of illicit drugs. Selective interventions are those aimed toward individuals who are members of a subgroup or population that is known to be at higher risk for a given disorder, for example, aiming interventions at teenagers to prevent drug abuse and drinking. Indicated interventions are for those individuals who exhibit a known risk factor, condition, or abnormality that identifies them as being at high risk for developing a disorder. Indicated interventions include providing education about alcoholism to young people whose parents are alcoholics or monitoring drug and alcohol use in people with depression or other commonly co-occurring psychiatric disorders. All three types of interventions are employed to prevent drug abuse and the effectiveness of various approaches is the subject of ongoing research.

TREATING ADDICTIVE DISORDERS

One of the most enduring myths about addiction is that treatment for these disorders is ineffective. Although addiction involves a complex interplay of biological, social, and individual factors that complicates treatment, the same can be said about the treatment for diabetes, hypertension, or asthma, which are also complicated by an interplay of disease severity, the individual's motivation and ability to control diet or exercise levels, social support, and other factors. Yet, there are important differences between addiction and these other illnesses in the perception of the public, insurance companies, and physicians. Few would argue that retreatment for diabetes, hypertension, or asthma indicates treatment failure, or that retreatment should be withheld from or denied to these patients when they relapse and their symptoms reoccur. Such an argument, however, is commonly made about addiction.

The general effectiveness of addiction treatment may be obscured by the tremendous variation in the types of services offered and in the amount of information available regarding the effectiveness of individual programs. In part, the variety reflects different approaches that have developed over time to address addiction to specific drugs (e.g., heroin vs. alcohol). In addition, not all strategies are possible to employ for specific addictions. For example, there are successful replacement pharmacotherapies available for herion and nicotine addiction (methadone and nicotine gum or patches), but not for alcohol or cocaine. Often, however, treatment approaches are based on underlying assumptions and viewpoints regarding the causes of addiction, ranging from addiction as a disease to addiction as a moral failure.

It is important to keep in mind that success or failure in treatment involves both treatment factors (e.g., setting, length, intensity) and patient factors (e.g., severity of addiction, presence of other psychiatric and medical conditions, social support, education, and readiness for change). The interaction of specific treatment factors with specific patient factors, often called patient-treatment matching, is one area of great interest in research. Ongoing research in a variety of disciplines, coupled with a better base of interdisciplinary and health services and treatment outcomes research, can be expected to improve the quality and availability of treatment for addiction and, thus, reduce the attendant individual and societal costs.

RECOMMENDATIONS

Education and Training

All secondary schools offer science courses, and many offer classes in psychology, sociology, and health education. The committee believes that strategies are needed to enhance the educational curricula in drug addiction. Students should be learning about the genetic and biological underpinnings of addiction, and how they interact with psychosocial and behavioral factors in the process of becoming addicted, overcoming addiction, and relapse. There is also a complementary need to improve the expertise of faculty so that well-qualified professionals who are capable of developing the necessary curricula are available to teach students about addicted individuals and addiction research.

The committee recommends that:

- **The U.S. Department of Education should provide incentives for schools to increase emphasis on the physiological and psychosocial aspects of drug abuse and addiction in science and health education classes at elementary, middle school, and high school levels; and**
- **Professional societies should facilitate expanding coverage of a science-based approach to understanding drug abuse and addiction at the**

university undergraduate level, especially in general psychology, sociology, and biology courses. Additional reviews should also be undertaken of related curricula in departments of social work, rehabilitation, and health education.

Graduate schools offer relatively few courses in substance abuse. A survey of American Psychological Association (APA)-approved graduate programs in clinical psychology, as well as graduate programs in sociology, and pharmacy programs, revealed that students receive only minimal training in drug abuse, although some disciplines are beginning to improve their curricula in the area of addiction. It appears that there are more opportunities for training in drug abuse counseling than in research-oriented programs, and these opportunities are primarily at a less advanced educational level. This lack of attention to addiction research in the curricula at the graduate school level may discourage students who are interested in the field.

The lack of instruction on drug abuse and addiction is a particular problem in medical schools. Less than one percent of curriculum time is spent on drug addiction in medical schools in the United States. The committee believes that the lack of emphasis on this important health and social issue is likely to convey to young medical professionals that this is not an important area of clinical work or research inquiry. Although opportunities in educational and training programs for addiction researchers exist, serious gaps remain. An effective medical training system must be both responsive to the differing needs of individuals at various stages of their careers and provide expertly trained professionals capable of addressing the health consequences related to addiction.

The committee recommends the following:

- **Accreditation and certifying entities [e.g., Liaison Committee on Medical Education (LCME), American Psychological Association (APA)] should review curricula in medical schools, and in psychology, social work, and nursing departments for the adequacy of drug addiction courses and should require basic competence in these areas for certification and recertification on medical specialty board examinations and in other relevant disciplines;**
- **Deans, administrators, and professional societies should undertake systematic evaluation of existing curricula to assess how they encourage or discourage training in addiction research and develop curricula tailored to different levels of schooling and specialty. Incentives should be provided to recruit and train faculty to teach courses in addiction research and to serve as role models.**

Mentors are needed at all stages of research training as well as for different groups of students, such as women and minorities. There is no single strategy that could increase and sustain the number and quality of mentors; several different efforts are needed.

To enable appropriate mentoring experiences, the committee recommends that:

- **Ph.D. programs in the behavioral and social sciences should be included among the degrees eligible for M.D./Ph.D. (MSTP) support;**
- **NIDA and NIAAA should increase the number of mentors by promoting interdisciplinary research through the establishment of funding mechanisms for mentoring teams composed of investigators from different disciplines in the Academic Centers of Excellence programs;**
- **NIDA and NIAAA should emphasize innovative mentoring programs through the K05, K07, and other K award mechanisms; and**
- **NIDA and NIAAA should consider reviving the Career Teacher Training Program.**

Although the focus of this report is on addiction research, the issues of treatment and research are often intertwined. Faculty who have expertise in treating addicted individuals can stimulate faculty who have expertise in conducting basic or applied research on addiction. Likewise, the availability and quality of treatment are dependent on innovative research findings. Furthermore, many graduate students, medical students, postdoctoral students, and medical residents will be exposed to the field of addiction research while being supervised in treatment settings.

The committee recommends that:

- **All treatment professionals should have some knowledge of basic neuroscience and how alcohol, nicotine, and other drugs work on brain pathways, influence behavior, and interact with diverse conditions. Treatment professionals should include physicians, nurses, clinical psychologists, social workers, drug abuse peer counselors, and other health care providers who work in conjunction with one another in treating patients with an addictive disease;**
- **Continuing education courses to update treatment professionals' knowledge base on addiction should be instituted systematically and widely; and**
- **Competence-based documentation of treatment professionals' knowledge base on addiction should be sought in licensing and recertification examinations.**

The committee identified several problems with the mechanisms that support careers in addiction research. These include insufficient numbers of traineeships and fellowships, insufficient research career development and sustaining awards, varying applicant success rates, and a low percentage of training support as a percentage of extramural funding. For example, fellowship training time is often insufficient for clinical researchers, who need to accommodate their clinical responsibilities with sufficient time for research training. Changes in this system need to be established as a government priority because there is limited support for career development from industry, universities, and private foundations.

Resources Needed for Young Investigators

Young investigators trained in the disciplines relevant to addiction research seek postdoctoral fellowships or salaried positions in universities, academic medical centers, or pharmaceutical companies. Those who seek academic careers usually apply for positions where the salary is at least partly secure, but their ability to conduct research is often dependent on research funding that has been obtained by a colleague (e.g., a senior researcher who is in charge of the postdoctoral training program) or funding that they must obtain by writing or assisting in the writing of a successful research grant application. The launching and sustained development of a research career is therefore dependent upon the availability of fellowship programs, research grants, and other mechanisms to support such careers.

To meet the challenges for developing careers in addiction research, the committee recommends that:

• **The number of research career development awards should be increased, greater flexibility in duration and time-to-start of awards should be provided, and the funding priority of such awards should be advanced;**

• **The use of the B/START (Behavioral Science Track Award for Rapid Transition) mechanism now at NIMH and NIDA to provide seed money for young investigators should be expanded;**

• **Programs for student-directed summer research should be established by NIDA and NIAAA;**

• **Industry and private foundations should cooperate with universities to provide supplemental funds for career development and research support of young investigators, especially during transition periods between awards, or to provide partial salary support for clinical researchers;**

• **Increases should be made in the percentage of NIDA and NIAAA extramural research funding spent on training programs to reach the NIH institute average (currently 5 percent to 6 percent), funds for which should *not* be redirected from the research budgets of these institutes;**

• **Jointly sponsored programs (e.g., government, industry, private foundations, academia) to support research training should be established** with clear roles and responsibilities for the participation of each institution; and

• NIDA and NIAAA should explore the possibility of providing bridging support for promising young investigators to assist in the transition from K01 and R29 to R01 funding.

To encourage clinical research on the problems of addiction, the committee recommends that:

• The federal government should establish a debt deferral or forgiveness program for scientists conducting clinical research in drug addiction or treating persons with drug abuse in publicly funded settings; and
• Federal funds should be made available from NIH, SAMSHA, HRSA, or AHCPR to provide training for primary care physicians (e.g., obstetricians, family physicians, and internists) to recognize, treat effectively, or refer patients with drug abuse problems.

In light of the recent advances in the field and the importance of collaborative and integrative research efforts to address the problems of addiction and relapse, the committee recommends that:

• Funding institutions, such as the government and private foundations, should develop program funding mechanisms (e.g., Requests for Applications [RFAs], annual conferences, symposia) to foster collaborative exchanges of information and research, such as the scientific breakthroughs that occur during drug development;
• Universities with faculty engaged in addiction research should undertake a comprehensive review of the support and resources available for collaborative efforts within and outside the university, particularly those collaborative efforts which involve multiple disciplines; administrators should develop a plan to share resources and facilities both within and across institutions and specify criteria for access;
• Funding agencies, such as the government and private foundations, should focus on new integrative opportunities (e.g., drug addiction etiology and medications) through using the combined strengths of the participating institutions, including government, industry, private foundations, multidisciplinary centers, and Academic Centers of Excellence;
• NIH should review the composition of Initial Review Groups (IRGs) to ensure that there is appropriate representation across necessary disciplines;
• NIDA and NIAAA should consider establishing additional mechanisms or expanding R03 awards for individual investigator awards that support innovative, high-risk, interdisciplinary research; and

• Additional sources of resources to increase and support integrative and collaborative efforts in addiction research should be considered by Congress. For example, the percentage of the budget of the White House Office of National Drug Control Policy earmarked for research should be increased substantially as part of a coordinated strategy to make drug abuse and addiction research a national priority.

Public Perceptions and Public Policy

Although there have been many scientific advances in our knowledge about drug addiction, the public's perceptions and understanding lag far behind. If the goal is to increase interest in and support for careers in addiction research, it is essential to communicate the current scientific knowledge base in an effective way to the public at large. Educating the public begins in schools and is carried further through the media and other mechanisms.

To help inform the public and build advocacy for destigmatizing addiction research, the committee recommends that:

• Public education campaigns should be based on an interdisciplinary view of addiction and emphasize treatment effectiveness, as well as include descriptions of the role of brain physiology and function (e.g., pain systems, anxiety circuits, mood systems, and behavioral and psychosocial aspects).

• Consumer and other advocacy groups should be encouraged to strengthen their focus on the need for research on the causes, prevention, and treatment of addictive disorders.

• Liaison relationships and joint activities should be explored among advocacy groups to increase public understanding of addictive disorders. Activities could include meetings of representatives of provider groups, state and local health departments, and established grassroots advocacy groups to develop cohesive, workable strategies to accomplish change.

All of these efforts will contribute to the long-term goals and strategies that the committee deems essential to resolve the broad problems found in this scientific area.

NOTES

1. One committee member, Dr. Satel, disagreed with this definition. She believes that, "The concept of addiction as a brain disease is somewhat limited and potentially misleading. Many workers find it more instructive to define addiction as a complex be-

havioral condition that is accompanied by organic changes in the brain but which is not inevitably sustained by them.

In conventional brain disorders such as schizophrenia or Parkinson's disease, symptoms of disturbed mentation and action are the result of brain pathology. In compulsive drug use, conversely, the brain changes are a result of that behavior. These changes, it is true, likely predispose to craving and rapid re-habituation in individuals who have been drug free, thus making them vulnerable to relapse. Yet it is important to emphasize that the course of addiction can be modified by its consequences and that biological urges can be overridden. The addiction as a brain disease model tends to obscure this clinical reality."

2. The class of opioids includes heroin, codeine, morphine, and synthetic opioids, while the stimulants include cocaine, amphetamine, methamphetamine, and methylphenidate.

1

Introduction

Every year, approximately half a million men, women, and children in the United States die from illnesses, unintentional injuries, and homicides attributed to the use of nicotine, alcohol, and illegal drugs (McGinnis and Foege, 1993). This represents one of every four deaths.

The economic consequences of drug addiction and abuse are staggering; their cost is estimated at more than $257 billion per year. Although legal drugs account for the vast majority of deaths and health-related costs, illegal drugs also have dramatic economic costs to governments and communities, including costs related to crime and crime prevention. Employers also share the burden of costs related to drug use in terms of increased worker's compensation, absenteeism, and lost productivity. The consequences of using nicotine, alcohol, and illegal drugs cut across every economic, social, racial, religious, and political stratum (IOM, 1990; OTA, 1994).

The problems of drug and alcohol abuse and addiction have been the focus of numerous reports over the past decade, including many from the Institute of Medicine (IOM) and the National Research Council (NRC). Although several of the IOM/NRC reports have focused on research opportunities and training issues across a variety of disciplines or pertinent to a specific federal agency (e.g., the National Institute on Drug Abuse [NIDA] or the National Institute on Alcohol Abuse and Alcoholism [NIAAA]), most were aimed toward audiences with research, clinical practice, or science policy backgrounds. One theme present in nearly all the IOM/NRC reports, however, is that addiction research is often perceived by the public and by policymakers as less important or less worthy than other types of biomedical research. Given the large public health and societal costs of addiction, after discussing the various reports, the IOM Board on Neuroscience and Behavioral Health (NBH) decided to examine this theme more closely, to assess the impact of the public perception about addiction research on the recruitment of talented young investigators into the field, and to examine specific career pathways in addiction research.

In July 1995, the IOM formed the Committee to Identify Strategies to Raise the Profile of Substance Abuse and Alcoholism Research with sponsorship from the W.M. Keck Foundation of Los Angeles. The major goals of the study were to identify strategies to increase the visibility of the important contributions of research on addiction, identify factors that may encourage and discourage the entry and career longevity of talented researchers in the field, and suggest ways to reduce any disincentives found.

The committee identified six areas that present challenges in the research and public arenas and developed strategies to address these challenges. These areas include:

- integrative and collaborative research,
- opportunities for education and training,
- funding stability and adequacy,
- public misunderstanding of addiction,
- stigma, and
- advocacy.

Where possible, the committee drew upon published literature and previous studies. However, given the limited literature on barriers to drug addiction research, the committee also sought information from experts within the field, government reports and agencies, professional organizations, and questionnaires sent to administrators, foundations, and accreditation organizations. In addition, the committee sponsored a workshop focused heavily on identifying existing barriers and discussing possible strategies to overcome them (Appendix A). Participants included junior and senior researchers inside and outside the field, administrators, policymakers, and representatives of industry and private foundations (Appendix B). The workshop included two plenary lectures (Appendixes C and D).

This report is the result of the committee's deliberations and represents an attempt to outline the challenges and opportunities in addiction research in a way that will be understandable to a somewhat different audience than previous IOM/NRC reports. Thus, this report is aimed at primary and secondary school educators and students, legislative aides and elected officials at all levels, and the media, as well as at college and early graduate students, graduate and medical school curricula developers, and federal agencies and foundations that fund training programs in the biomedical sciences.

DEFINITIONS AND CONCEPTS

There is much confusion and controversy in both the scientific and lay literature regarding the terms used in addiction research, including "addiction," "abuse," and even what should be called a drug. The effect of multiple definitions and confusing terminology should not be underestimated; the committee itself struggled with these controversies.

One of the debates in the field is whether addiction is best defined as a disorder, a chronic disease, a complex set of symptoms, or a behavioral condition. This and other IOM committees have defined drug addiction as a **brain disease** similar to other chronic, relapsing conditions, such as heart disease and diabetes, and manifested by a complex set of behaviors that are the result of genetic, biological, psychosocial, and environmental interactions (IOM, 1995, 1996).[1]

Medical diagnostic systems have defined addiction as compulsive use of a drug that is not medically necessary, accompanied by impairment in health or social functioning (APA, 1994; WHO, 1992).[2] The term "substance dependence" is used by these classification systems as equivalent to addiction, but the term dependence is often confused with other aspects of addiction. For example, it is sometimes considered to be synonymous with the term "tolerance," a physiological process in which repeated doses of a drug over time elicit a progressively decreasing effect and the person requires higher or more frequent doses of the drug to achieve the same results. There are situations in which tolerance can be present in the absence of compulsive craving; for example, a person being treated with morphine for chronic pain. However, few such individuals become pathologically addicted; once treatment is no longer needed, they do not engage in compulsive drug-seeking behavior.

---

[1]One committee member, Dr. Satel, disagreed with this definition. She believes that, "The concept of addiction as a brain disease is somewhat limited and potentially misleading. Many workers find it more instructive to define addiction as a complex behavioral condition that is accompanied by organic changes in the brain but which is not inevitably sustained by them.

In conventional brain disorders such as schizophrenia or Parkinson's disease, symptoms of disturbed mentation and action are the result of brain pathology. In compulsive drug use, conversely, the brain changes are a result of that behavior. These changes, it is true, likely predispose to craving and rapid re-habituation in individuals who have been drug free, thus making them vulnerable to relapse. Yet it is important to emphasize that the course of addiction can be modified by its consequences and that biological urges can be overridden. The addiction as a brain disease model tends to obscure this clinical reality."

[2]Drug use is not defined in either system as a medical disorder. Abuse, or harmful use, is mentioned in these systems as being characterized by higher use accompanied by legal, social, or interpersonal problems.

Almost any discussion of addiction causes controversy. There has been a long and tortuous history in the development of our concepts of addiction based on changing political and social environments and on the legal status of the specific drugs themselves (see Appendix E). As the medical model of opioid addiction became accepted, the term addiction or "addict" was thought to carry a social stigma that undermined attempts to cast the problem as a disease and thereby to bolster more humane treatment of persons with addictive disorders. The term "dependence" seemed to lack such stigma and therefore it was applied to a broader range of problems (e.g., alcohol, nicotine, caffeine). Yet, dependence seems to many a loosely defined term that carries a connotation of some type of character flaw or lack of will.

Certainly there are psychological and cognitive underpinnings of addiction and many people are able to quit using drugs without medical or other types of interventions. However, these individuals nevertheless must struggle for months and sometimes years to overcome strong physiological (e.g., withdrawal symptoms) and motivational (e.g., drug craving) disturbances during recovery from addiction.

The application of the term "addiction" itself has been problematic in that it has tended, until recently, to be applied more frequently to illegal drugs than to legal ones. Interestingly, amidst the current legal and political struggles about smoking and nicotine, addiction has become the term of choice of those working to emphasize the physiological effects of nicotine. In the popular press and in colloquial language, the terms "addict" and "junkie" are applied to everything from chocolate to television.

A central tenet of this report is that addiction may occur as a consequence of using many different types of drugs or substances, some of which are legal and socially acceptable and some of which are illegal. For example, all of the following are potentially addictive drugs: alcohol, nicotine, caffeine, heroin and other opioids, cocaine, and amphetamines. These drugs may lead to physiological dependence and tolerance or a withdrawal syndrome when the drug is abruptly discontinued, or both. Further, the terms "addiction" and "dependence" are used interchangeably in their scientific sense to denote drug-seeking behavior involving compulsive use of high doses of one or more drugs for no clear medical indication, resulting in substantial impairment of health and social functioning.

CLASSIFICATION OF DRUGS

A drug is any chemical agent, other than a food, that affects biological function and is typically used in humans or other animals to prevent or treat a disease. A psychotropic drug is one that acts in the brain to alter mood, thought processes, or behavior (Goldstein, 1994).

Throughout the years, several typologies have been developed to classify different drug agents. In 1965, the World Health Organization (WHO) identified a typology of drug dependence based on seven classes of substances that were widely abused (Eddy et al., 1965). The current *Diagnostic and Statistical Manual of the American Psychiatric Association (DSM-IV)* has defined 11 classes of substances that may be part of a substance abuse *disorder* (APA, 1994). Seven families of addictive drugs that together comprise the drug abuse problem have been classified by Goldstein (1994), distinguished from one another on the basis of chemistry, behavioral effects, and the likelihood of addiction developing. Table 1.1 provides a classification that combines specific aspects of these three definitional frameworks. It lists nine classes of drugs, in order of their overall prevalence of use (highest to lowest) in the United States:

1. caffeine;
2. alcohol;
3. nicotine;
4. depressants, barbiturates, benzodiazepines;
5. marijuana and hashish;
6. opioids;
7. stimulants (cocaine, amphetamine, and related drugs);
8. hallucinogens; and
9. inhalants.

This classification system groups addictive and abusable drugs by functional or behavioral activity, independently of proposed receptor effects or mechanisms of action. It differs from the "seven families" classification by separating alcohol and related drugs into three different categories: alcohol, inhalants, and barbiturates. It differs from the *DSM-IV* by combining hallucinogens and phencyclidine (PCP) into one category, and eliminating the categories of "polysubstances" and "other" drugs.

The focus of this report is on four major classes of drugs: nicotine, alcohol, opioids, and stimulants.[3] These are emphasized because they have the greatest social and economic impact on society. In addition, the use of these drugs causes or contributes to many life-threatening disorders, including cirrhosis, AIDS, and cancer. The term "drug" is used in its generic sense to encompass all four substances, but where it is appropriate and necessary to be specific, reference is made to the specific drug or class of drugs.

---

[3]The class of opioids includes heroin, codeine, morphine, and synthetic opioids, while the stimulants include cocaine, amphetamine, methamphetamine, and methylphenidate.

ORGANIZATION OF THE REPORT

In the last few years, a great deal of progress has been made in the science of addiction and in treatment research (including improvements in diagnostic criteria) and development and evaluation of a wide range of treatments (including FDA approval of medications for treatment of opioid, alcohol, and nicotine dependence). To determine how to raise the profile of addiction research and attract the best possible researchers to the field, this scientific progress needs to be considered in light of the prevalence and costs of addiction, the current investments made in addiction research, and the gaps in research and resources.

The first part of this report provides an overview of what is currently known about drug abuse and addiction. Chapter 2 summarizes the economic costs resulting from addiction to nicotine, alcohol, and illegal drugs, and the funding investments in addiction research made by the federal government and the private sector compared to research funding for other chronic diseases. Chapter 3 describes the contributions of basic neurobiology to the understanding of drug addiction, and Chapter 4 gives an overview of research into the psychosocial aspects of addiction and strategies to prevent drug abuse and addiction. Chapter 5 is focused on the science base of drug treatment. In these three chapters, some promising research areas for the future are noted, but no formal recommendations are made. Another recent report from the IOM, *Pathways of Addiction*, presented recommendations for these research areas and for research on the effects of criminal justice approaches to prevent or decrease drug abuse (IOM, 1996). Thus, Chapters 2, 3, 4, and 5 of the present report are intended to provide a broad description of the richness of research on addictive disorders.

The remaining chapters of the present report examine what is needed to develop a talented cadre of researchers and educate the public about addiction research. These chapters identify specific barriers to progress and offer recommendations and suggestions for strategies that may lessen the impact of these barriers. Chapter 6 identifies critical issues regarding the education and training of future addiction researchers, including science curricula in schools and colleges, graduate schools, and medical schools, as well as issues of mentoring and the need for interdisciplinary training. Chapter 7 examines some of the resource infrastructure and funding levels for addiction research, particularly those available for new researchers. This chapter also assesses the funding levels of research grants in addiction compared to research on other diseases and delineates some of the barriers that may hinder some health professionals from pursuing careers in addiction research and prevent progress in some areas of research. Chapter 8 describes how public perceptions influence education and public policies, and how these perceptions may inhibit improvement of the public's understanding of addiction.

TABLE 1.1 Classification of Abusive and Addictive Drugs

Class	Description
Caffeine	Produces wakefulness, mild central nervous system (CNS) and cardiovascular stimulation. Mild tolerance, dependence following chronic use.
Alcohol (ethyl alcohol, ethanol)	Produces dose-dependent relaxation, disinhibition, mild euphoria, inebriation, intoxication, CNS depression (similar to CNS depressants), liver damage. Significant tolerance and dependence-withdrawal following chronic use; intense craving; alcoholism.
Nicotine	Present in all forms of tobacco. Produces mild CNS and cardiovascular stimulation. Tolerance and dependence-withdrawal following chronic use; intense craving; nicotine addiction.
Depressants (sedatives, hypnotics, anxiolytics): barbiturates, methaqualone, diazepam, and other benzodiazepines	Produce dose-dependent relaxation, disinhibition, mild euphoria, inebriation, intoxication, CNS depression. Significant tolerance and dependence-withdrawal following chronic use; craving; addiction.
Cannabinoids (marijuana, hashish): tetrahydrocanna-binol (THC)	Produce dose-dependent relaxation, disinhibition; alterations of mood, emotion, and behavior; inebriation, intoxication. Mild tolerance; little or no withdrawal.
Opiates (opioids) and related analgesics: heroin, codeine, morphine, synthetic opioids	Produce dose-dependent analgesia, euphoria, disinhibition, anesthesia, CNS depression. Significant tolerance and dependence-withdrawal following chronic use; intense craving; opioid addiction.
Stimulants: cocaine, amphetamine, methamphet-amine, methylphenidate	Produce dose-dependent mild-strong CNS stimulation, behavioral hyperactivity, adverse cardiovascular effects, euphoria. Tolerance and dependence-withdrawal following chronic use; intense craving; addiction.
Hallucinogens: lysergic acid diethylamide (LSD), mescaline, psilocybin, dimethyltryptamine (DMT), dimethoxymethylamphet-amine (DOM), MDA, MDMA ("ecstasy"), phencyclidine (PCP; "angel dust"), ketamine	Symptoms vary depending on which drug: visual distortions, hallucinations, mood changes, arousal, euphoria, anxiety, agitation, emotional withdrawal, thought disturbances, aggressive behavior, panic, catatonia. Mild tolerance with chronic use; little or no withdrawal.

continues

TABLE 1.1 Continued

Class	Description
Inhalants: solvents, aerosols, acetone, benzene, nitrous oxide, amyl nitrate	Produce dose-dependent relaxation, mild euphoria, dizziness, disinhibition, inebriation, intoxication, anesthesia, CNS depression, liver damage, cardiovascular depression.

SOURCES: APA (1994), Eddy et al. (1965), Goldstein (1994), O'Brien (1996), and OTA (1994).

REFERENCES

APA (American Psychiatric Association). 1994. *Diagnostic and Statistical Manual of Mental Disorders: DSM-IV.* 4th Edition. Washington, DC: American Psychiatric Association.

Eddy NB, Halbach H, Isbell H, Seevers MH. 1965. Drug dependence: Its significance and characteristics. *Bulletin of the World Health Organization* 32:721–733.

Goldstein A. 1994. *Addiction: From Biology to Policy.* New York: W.H. Freeman and Company.

IOM (Institute of Medicine). 1990. *Treating Drug Problems.* Vol. 1. Washington, DC: National Academy Press.

IOM. 1995. *The Development of Medications for the Treatment of Opiate and Cocaine Addictions: Issues for the Government and Private Sector.* Washington, DC: National Academy Press.

IOM. 1996. *Pathways of Addiction: Opportunities in Drug Abuse Research.* Washington, DC: National Academy Press.

McGinnis JM, Foege WH. 1993. Actual causes of death in the United States. *Journal of the American Medical Association* 270(18):2207–2212.

O'Brien CP. 1996. Drug addiction and drug abuse. In: Hardman JG, Limbird LE, Molinoff PB, Rudden RW, Gilman AG, eds. *Goodman and Goodman's The Pharmacological Basis of Therapeutics.* 9th Edition. New York: McGraw-Hill. Pp. 557–577.

OTA (Office of Technology Assessment). 1994. *Technologies for Understanding and Preventing Substance Abuse and Addiction.* OTA-EHR-597. Washington, DC: U.S. Government Printing Office.

WHO (World Health Organization). 1992. *International Statistical Classification of Diseases and Related Health Problems.* 10th Revision. Geneva: World Health Organization.

2

Prevalence, Costs, and Investments

Drug abuse has been called the nation's number one public health problem (Institute for Health Policy, 1993). One of every $12 of the nation's personal health care expenditures is spent on prevention, diagnosis, and treatment of people suffering from addictive diseases. Illicit drugs, such as opioids and stimulants, alcohol, and nicotine are responsible for debilitating illnesses and diseases, premature deaths, and the overburdening of the medical, social services, and criminal justice systems. This chapter provides a brief overview of the prevalence and measurable economic consequences of addictive drugs and the investments currently being made in research, prevention, treatment, and law enforcement.

PREVALENCE

During high school, almost every child in America confronts the choice of whether to use illicit drugs, drink alcohol, and smoke cigarettes, and many children take their first drug even before entering high school. Individuals who reach age 20 without having used marijuana, smoked cigarettes, or abused alcohol are unlikely ever to do so. The risk of cocaine use peaks between the ages of 21 and 24 and tapers off by age 30 (Chen and Kandel, 1995). Thus, drug addiction can be viewed as a pediatric disorder that becomes a major problem in late adolescence and early adulthood. As a result, many prevention efforts are aimed at early and experimental drug exposure. Although many people who occasionally use illicit drugs, drink alcohol, or smoke do not experience problems, the risk of addiction increases with heavier or more frequent consumption.

Illicit Drugs

In 1995, the Substance Abuse and Mental Health Service Administration's (SAMHSA's) National Household Survey on Drug Abuse estimated that 12.8 million Americans used at least one illicit drug during the past month, constituting 6.1 percent of the population 12 years old or older—a dramatic decrease from 1979 when the number of current illicit drug users was at its highest level of 25 million or 14 percent of the population (SAMHSA, 1996a). Although the estimated number of users has remained at approximately the same level since 1992, rates of drug use show substantial variation by age with the greatest increases of use occurring among young people ages 16–20 (SAMHSA, 1996a) (see Figure 2.1). According to the 1996 National Institute on Drug Abuse's (NIDA) Monitoring the Future Study, 24.6 percent of high school seniors used at least one illicit drug in the past month—a slight increase since 1995 (23.8 percent), reflecting the continued rise in illicit drug use by teenagers since 1992 when the rate was at the lowest percentage of 14.4 (Johnston et al., 1997).

In regard to ethnicity, gender, geography, education, and employment, the rates of current illicit drug use in 1995 varied as follows (SAMHSA, 1996a):

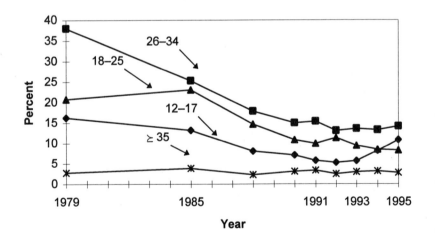

FIGURE 2.1 Past month illicit drug use by age: 1979–1995. SOURCE: SAMHSA (1996a).

• Ethnicity—The rate of current illicit drug use for African Americans (7.9 percent) remained somewhat higher than for Caucasians, (6.0 percent) and Hispanics (5.1 percent). However, among youths (ages 12–17) the rates of use are about the same across the three groups. Most current illicit drug users (have used at least one illicit drug in the past month) are Caucasian representing 75 percent of all users (9.6 million); African Americans make up 15 percent (1.9 million), and Hispanics 8 percent (1.0 million). Although in selected age groups and with specific kinds of drugs there is an increased variability among different ethnic groups, the statistics rebut the prevailing racial stereotypes that minorities are the most prevalent users of illicit drugs. Among Native American populations, the survey literature of high school students indicates that, on average, rates of lifetime use and abuse of drugs, including alcohol, are higher among Native American than non-Native American youths (Libran and Smart, 1982; May, 1996; Winfree and Griffiths, 1985; Winfree et al., 1989). However, it is also noted that nonreservation Native American youths have higher rates of drug use compared to those living on reservations. These surveys present only averaged data from a variety of schools and locations and it is important to note that there is substantial variation among different Native American communities and tribal groups.

• Gender—Men continue to have higher rates of current illicit drug use than women (7.8 percent vs. 4.5 percent).

• Geography—Current illicit drug use rates ranged from 7.8 percent in the Western region of the United States to 4.9 in the Northeast; there was little difference in rates of use in large metropolitan areas, small metropolitan areas, and rural areas.

• Education—Illicit drug use rates remain highly correlated with educational status; among 18- to 34-year-olds, those who had not completed high school had the highest rate of use (15.4 percent), while college graduates had the lowest (5.9 percent). However, lifetime prevalence rates (i.e., having tried illicit drugs at least once in their life) are equal regardless of educational status.

• Employment—Current employment status is also highly correlated with rates of illicit drug use. In 1995, 14.3 percent of unemployed adults (age 18 and older) were current illicit drug users, compared to 5.5 percent of full-time employed adults. Seventy-one percent of all current illicit drug users age 18 and older (7.4 million adults) were employed, including 5.4 million full-time workers and 1.9 million part-time workers.

Alcohol

The number of Americans age 12 and older who had used alcohol in the past month was estimated at 111 million (52 percent of the population) in 1995. Of those 111 million, 32 million engaged in binge drinking (5 or more drinks on at least one occasion in the past month), including approximately 11 million who are considered heavy drinkers consuming 5 or more drinks per occasion on

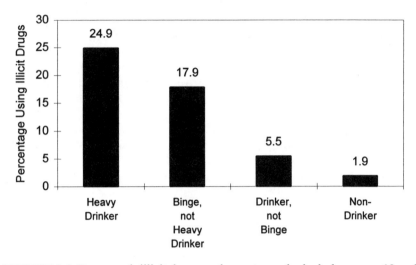

FIGURE 2.2 Past month illicit drug use, by past month alcohol use, age 12 and older, 1995. SOURCE: SAMHSA (1996a).

5 or more days in the past 30 days (SAMHSA, 1996a). Excessive alcohol con-sumption is responsible for more than 100,000 deaths per year in the United States (Doyle, 1996). Accidents—the fifth leading cause of death for all ages—accounted for 34.1 percent of all deaths, most due to drunk driving (Doyle, 1996; NCHS, 1996).

According to the National Household Survey on Drug Abuse, alcohol use may act as a gateway to using illicit drugs due to their strong association with each other. In 1995, 25 percent of the 11 million heavy drinkers were also cur-rent illicit drug users compared to only 1.9 percent of nondrinkers who reported having used illicit drugs in the past month (SAMHSA, 1996a) (see Figure 2.2).

In regard to age, ethnicity, gender, geography, and education, the rates of alcohol use in 1995 varied as follows (SAMHSA, 1996a):

• Age—Of the 111 million Americans who currently use alcohol, 10 million were under the age of 21; 4.4 million were binge drinkers, including 1.7 million heavy users. Young adults ages 18–25 were the most likely to binge or drink heavily.

• Ethnicity—Caucasians continue to have the highest rates of alcohol use at 56 percent, while rates for African Americans and Hispanics were 45 percent and 41 percent respectively. Binge use of alcohol was highest among Hispanics at 17.2 percent followed closely by Caucasians at 16.6 percent; African Ameri-cans had the lowest binge rate at 11.2 percent. Heavy use showed no statistically significant differences by ethnicity. Among adult Native Americans, studies show significant variations in prevalence of drinking from one tribal group to another. These studies have concluded that adult prevalence of alcohol abuse is lower in some tribes than the average U.S. general population rate while other tribes exhibit similar or higher rates than U.S. averages (May, 1989; May and Smith, 1988; Welty et al., 1995; Whittaker, 1982).

• Gender—Sixty percent of men were past month alcohol users while the figure for women was 45 percent; men were also much more likely than women to be binge drinkers (23.8 percent vs. 8.5 percent) and heavy drinkers (9.4 percent vs. 2.0 percent).

• Geography—Rates of past month alcohol use were 56 percent in large metropolitan areas, 52 percent in small metropolitan areas, and 46 percent in nonmetropolitan areas; there was little variation in binge and heavy alcohol use rates among the areas.

• Education—In contrast to the pattern for illicit drug use, the higher the educational level, the more likely was the current use of alcohol; in 1995, 68 percent of adults with college degrees were current drinkers compared to only 42 percent of those having less than a high school education. However, although the rate of binge drinking was similar across educational levels, 7.1 percent of adults who had not completed high school were heavy drinkers compared to 3.7 percent of adults who had completed college.

Nicotine

In 1995, 61 million Americans were current smokers, indicating a smoking rate of 29 percent for the population age 12 and older. An additional 6.9 million Americans were current users of smokeless tobacco (SAMHSA, 1996a). Current users of tobacco were more likely to be heavy drinkers and use illicit drugs compared to nonsmokers, thus highlighting the role of tobacco products as another gateway substance. In regard to age, ethnicity, gender, geography, and education, the rates varied in 1995 as follows (SAMHSA, 1996a):

• Age—Almost 4.5 million youths ages 12–17 (20 percent) were current smokers in 1995; those who smoked were approximately 8 times more likely to use illicit drugs and 11 times more likely to drink heavily as nonsmoking youths. In spite of the demonstrated health risks associated with smoking, prevalence rates among young people remain high. Since 1975, cigarettes have consistently been the substance that the greatest number of high school students use on a daily basis (Johnston et al., 1997).

• Ethnicity—No significant differences in smoking rates by ethnicity were established. Smokeless tobacco use, however, was more prevalent among Caucasians (3.9 percent) compared to African Americans or Hispanics (1.3 percent and 1.2 percent respectively).

• Gender—Men had somewhat higher rates of smoking compared to women, while the rate of smokeless tobacco use was significantly higher for men than for women (6.2 percent vs. 0.6 percent); over 90 percent of smokeless tobacco users were men in 1995.

• Geography—Smoking rates were 27 percent in large metropolitan areas, 28 percent in small metropolitan areas, and 33 percent in nonmetropolitan areas.

• Education—Thirty-seven percent of adults who had not completed high school smoked cigarettes compared to only 17 percent of college graduates.

Overall Trends in Illicit Drug, Alcohol, and Nicotine Use

Although the use among adults of addictive legal and illegal drugs has declined in recent years, there is no guarantee that these trends will continue. Smoking began to decline in the mid-1960s, illicit drug use in the late 1970s, and alcohol consumption in the mid-1980s. These declines may be attributed to increased awareness of the health risks of drug, alcohol, and nicotine use; more governmental involvement in prevention, intervention, and treatment efforts; and the development of a few grassroots efforts and coalitions (e.g., Mothers Against Drunk Driving, Americans for Nonsmokers' Rights) directed at reducing substance use and abuse and its negative consequences (Institute for Health Policy, 1993). Additional research on prevention and reduction of drug use, as well as continued tracking of drug use trends, is essential to maintaining and reducing the current levels of use.

TABLE 2.1 Trends in Past Month Use of Marijuana, Alcohol, and Cigarettes by 8th Graders, 10th Graders, and High School Seniors, 1992–1996

Drug and Age Group	1992	1993	1994	1995	1996
Marijuana					
8th graders	3.7	5.1	7.8	9.1	11.3
10th graders	8.1	10.9	15.8	17.2	20.4
High school seniors	11.9	15.5	19.0	21.2	21.9
Alcohol					
8th graders	26.1	26.2	25.5	24.6	26.2
10th graders	39.9	38.2	39.2	38.8	65.0
High school seniors	51.3	51.0	50.1	51.3	50.8
Cigarettes					
8th graders	15.5	16.7	18.6	19.1	21.0
10th graders	21.5	24.7	25.4	27.9	30.4
High school seniors	27.8	29.9	31.2	33.5	34.0

SOURCE: Johnston et al. (1997).

Illicit drug and nicotine use among youth shows a different and worrisome pattern. The proportion of young people between the ages of 12 and 17 who used illicit drugs in the previous month decreased from a peak of 16 percent in 1979 to a low of 5 percent in 1992, but then doubled to 11 percent in 1995 (SAMHSA, 1996a). Rates of smoking have also increased recently among teenagers. Since 1992, the percentage of high school seniors who smoke (as reported in the past 30 days) has increased from 27.8 percent to 34 percent in 1996 (Johnston et al., 1997). Trends in past month use of marijuana, alcohol, and cigarette use for 8th and 10th graders, and high school seniors for 1992–1996 are shown in Table 2.1. Of special note is that despite the overall lower smoking rates among African-American youths, the rate of smoking among young African-American males has doubled in recent years, from 14 percent in 1991 to 28 percent in 1995 (MMWR, 1996).

ECONOMIC COSTS OF ADDICTION

Estimating the Cost of Drug Abuse in the United States

Individuals who use and abuse illicit drugs, alcohol, and cigarettes have disproportionately high use of medical services and impose large costs on the economy and on the legal and criminal justice systems. Many studies of illicit drug, alcohol, and nicotine addiction have estimated the costs to the United States for addiction to each of these drugs both individually and collectively (Berry and Bowland, 1977; Cruze et al., 1981; Harwood et al., 1984; *MMWR*, 1994; OTA, 1985; Rice, 1993; Rice et al., 1986, 1990, 1991a–c, 1992; Shultz et al., 1991a,b). Estimates vary as a result of different data sets, different assumptions, and different methods of calculation. In 1990,[1] it was estimated that the abuse of illicit drugs, alcohol, and nicotine cost society approximately $257 billion (see Table 2.2). The economic cost to society was measured in terms of the *direct* medical care expenditures for treatment of patients suffering from the adverse health effects of use of these drugs, *indirect* costs associated with loss of earnings due to reduced or lost productivity (morbidity) and premature death (mortality), and *other related* costs (i.e., nonhealth care costs such as those associated with the criminal and social welfare systems).

---

[1]The year 1990 is used as the base year because it is the most recent for which the total costs to society of drug addiction have been estimated.

TABLE 2.2 Estimated Economic Costs of Illicit Drug, Alcohol, and Nicotine Abuse, 1990 (millions of dollars)

Type of Cost	Illicit Drugs	Alcohol	Nicotine
Total	$66,873	$98,623	$91,269
Core Costs	14,602	80,763	91,269
Direct	3,197	10,512	39,130
Mental health/specialty organizations	867	3,469	—
Short stay hospitals	1,889	4,589	21,072
Office-based physicians	88	240	12,251
Other professional services	32	329	—[a]
Prescription drugs	—	—	1,469
Nursing homes	—	1,095	3,858
Home health services	—	—	480
Support costs	321	790	—
Indirect	11,405	70,251	52,139
Morbidity[b]	7,997	36,627	6,603
Mortality[c]	3,408	33,624	45,536
Other Related Costs	45,989	15,771	—
Direct	18,043	10,436	—
Crime	18,035	5,807	—
Motor vehicle crashes	—	3,876	—
Fire destruction	—	633	—
Social welfare administration	8	120	—
Indirect	27,946	5,335	—
Victims of crime	1,042	576	—
Incarceration	7,813	4,759	—
Crime careers	19,091	—	—
AIDS	6,282	—	—
Fetal alcohol syndrome	—	2,089	—

NOTE: 1990 costs for illicit drugs and alcohol abuse are based on socioeconomic indexes applied to 1985 estimates (Rice et al., 1990). Cigarette direct smoking costs are deflated from 1993 direct cost estimates (MMWR, 1994) and cigarette indirect costs are from Rice (1992).

[a]Amounts spent for other professional services are included in office-based physicians.
[b]Value of goods and services lost by individuals unable to perform their usual activities because of drug abuse or unable to perform them at a level of full effectiveness (Rice et al., 1990).
[c]Present value of future earnings lost, illicit drugs and alcohol discounted at 6 percent, nicotine discounted at 4 percent.

SOURCE: MMWR (1994), Rice (1992, 1995 [personal communication]), Rice et al. (1990).

In 1990, the total economic cost estimates varied widely for each substance, with alcohol and nicotine inflicting the greatest direct and indirect costs (see Figure 2.3). Nicotine addiction comprised almost three-fourths (74 percent) of the total substance-related direct costs of $52.8 billion. Alcohol accounted for 20 percent, and illegal drugs for the remaining 6 percent. In regard to morbidity costs, alcohol constituted 72 percent of the $51 billion spent while nicotine made up 55 percent of the $82.6 billion spent on mortality costs. Illegal drugs made up 17 percent of the morbidity costs, 4 percent of the mortality costs, but 75 percent of the $61.8 billion for other related costs (other related costs are not available for nicotine).

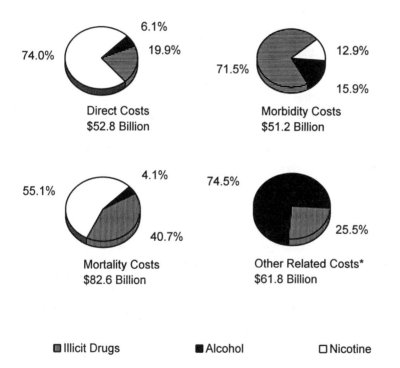

Direct Costs
$52.8 Billion

Morbidity Costs
$51.2 Billion

Mortality Costs
$82.6 Billion

Other Related Costs*
$61.8 Billion

▦ Illicit Drugs   ■ Alcohol   □ Nicotine

FIGURE 2.3 Economic costs of addiction by type of cost and drug, 1990. *Estimates for nicotine were not available. SOURCES: IOM (1995) and Rice (1995).

BOX 2.1
Estimating the Cost of Drug Abuse in New York City

The Center on Addiction and Substance Abuse at Columbia University (CASA) published a comprehensive study detailing how drug abuse and addiction in New York City cost more than $20 billion in 1994. They estimated $5.1 billion in health care; $4.9 billion in productivity lost from the city's economy; $4.1 billion in police, courts, prisons and the rest of the criminal justice system; $3.5 billion in public and private social services including welfare, food stamps, and foster care; $1.6 billion in increased insurance, security and workers' compensation costs to business; and $835 million in property costs. Only $735 million (3.7 percent) of the $20 billion was spent on treating drug abuse and addiction, and only $80 million (0.4 percent) was spent to prevent it; the vast majority of the $20 billion ($19.2 billion) paid for the consequences of the problem (CASA, 1996). The authors believe that the $20 billion estimate for the cost of drug abuse and addiction for New York City, although staggering, may be underestimated by 10 to 15 percent because of under-reporting in household surveys, unreported crimes, inadequate health records, and the inability to quantify education costs (CASA, 1996).

An example of the impact of the high economic costs of drug abuse in one U.S. city (New York City) is described in Box 2.1.

Comparison of Drug Addiction Costs with Costs of Other Diseases

The total cost to society of alcohol, nicotine, and illicit drug abuse totaled $257 billion in 1990, which was higher than the costs of other highly prevalent and costly diseases, such as mental disorders, diabetes, heart disease, cancer, stroke, and AIDS (see Table 2.3). For example, total costs of mental disorders in 1990 were estimated to be $148 billion, diabetes costs were $137 billion (does not include other related costs), heart diseases costs were $133 billion (does not include other related costs), and cancer costs were $96 billion (does not include other related costs). It is important to note that the costs of heart diseases and cancer include the costs of persons who are treated or die as a result of nicotine-related illness, so there is overlap between these categories.

INVESTMENTS

Investing in research focused on the causes, prevention, and treatment of addictive behavior, as well as in training new researchers and clinicians participating in the field, ultimately enables society to adequately assist those addicted,

TABLE 2.3 Costs of Illness for Selected Diseases and Conditions (billions of dollars)

Disease	Year	Total	Direct	Indirect	Other Related[a]
Drug Addiction, Total	1990	256.8	52.8	133.8	61.8
Alcohol[b]	1990	98.6	10.5	70.3	15.8
Illicit Drugs[c]	1990	66.9	3.2	11.4	46.0
Nicotine (IOM, 1995; Rice, 1995)	1990	91.3	39.1	52.1	n/a
Mental Disorders, Total[d]	1990	147.8	67.0	74.8	6.0
Anxiety disorders	1990	46.5	10.7	35.4	0.4
Schizophrenia	1990	32.5	17.3	12.0	3.2
Affective disorders	1990	30.4	19.2	9.9	1.3
Other disorders (Rice and Miller, 1996)	1990	38.4	19.7	17.6	1.1
Diabetes (Varmus, 1995)	1992	137.1	91.1	46.6	n/a
Heart Diseases (NHLBI, 1994)	1993	133.2	71.9	61.3	n/a
Cancer (all sites) (Varmus, 1995)	1990	96.1	27.5	68.7	n/a
Stroke (NHLBI, 1994)	1993	35.5	21.9	13.6	n/a
AIDS (Varmus, 1995)	1992	n/a	10.3	n/a	n/a

NOTE: 1990 is used as the base year because it is the most recent date for which the total costs to society of substance addiction and mental disorders have been estimated. For comparison, cost estimates for diabetes, heart diseases, cancer, stroke, and AIDS are based on the years listed closest to 1990. However, given that the cost estimates were calculated by different sources, the numbers may not be directly comparable and serve only to provide an overview of the estimated cost of each illness to society. It should also be noted that when other related costs are subtracted from the total for drug addition, the cost ($186.6 billion) still exceeds all other estimates.

n/a = not available.

[a]Other related costs include crime, victims of crime, incarceration, motor vehicle crashes, fire destruction, and social welfare administration.
[b]Total includes costs of fetal alcohol syndrome (FAS).
[c]Total includes costs of AIDS.
[d]Includes costs of adverse health effects of drugs.

SOURCES: IOM (1995), NHLBI (1994), Rice (1995), Rice and Miller (1996), and Varmus (1995).

prevent abuse and dependence, and reduce adverse individual and social consequences and associated costs (IOM, 1996). Adverse health consequences of addiction to illicit drugs, alcohol, or nicotine include increased transmission of human immunodeficiency virus (HIV), tuberculosis, morbidity, and mortality due to accidents, fetal alcohol syndrome (FAS), cirrhosis, and cancer—all of which exact an enormous social and economic burden on society. The total overall cost of illicit drug, alcohol, and nicotine use and abuse is approximately $257 billion (in 1990) exceeding the annual estimated cost of cancer ($104 billion in 1997) and coronary heart disease ($91 billion in 1997) (AHA, 1997; ACS, 1997; Rice 1995).

The federal government plays a leading role in providing funding for research, prevention, treatment, and law enforcement. In 1996, the federal government spent $13.5 billion dollars on drug abuse, with $609.2 million (4.5 percent of the total) for research and development. In comparison, $9.0 billion (67 percent of the FY 1996 budget) was spent on criminal justice programs; $2.6 billion (19 percent) on treatment of drug abuse and $1.4 billion (10 percent) on prevention efforts (see Figure 2.4) (ONDCP, 1997).

In 1996, the National Institute on Drug Abuse (NIDA) and National Institute on Alcohol Abuse and Alcoholism (NIAAA) spent a total of $504 million on drug addiction research and $16 million on training of drug addiction researchers (NIH, 1997). However, in comparison, the National Heart, Lung, and Blood Institute spent $983 million for research and $48 million for training, and the National Cancer Institute spent $1.215 billion for cancer research and $39 million to train cancer researchers in 1995 alone. Against this discrepancy, both NIDA and NIAAA continue to expand their research efforts in providing a greater understanding of the problem of addiction and how addiction can be prevented and treated; total NIDA and NIAAA investment in research and training for 1996 represent a 52 percent and 38 percent increase over 1990 spending levels (see Table 2.4 and 2.5).

The Substance Abuse and Mental Health Services Administration (SAMHSA), which includes a Center for Substance Abuse Prevention (CSAP) and a Center for Substance Abuse Treatment (CSAT), was created by statute in 1992 to focus on services for addiction and training of practitioners and others (e.g., counselors, program administrators) involved in addiction rather than on research. As part of the National Institutes of Health, NIDA, NIAAA, and the National Institute of Mental Health focus entirely on research related to basic research, prevention, diagnosis, treatment, and health services research, as well as on the training of researchers and clinicians interested in doing addiction research. SAMHSA and its centers provide funding for demonstration projects to prevent and treat drug abuse, but these projects have not been rigorously evaluated. In FY 1995, CSAP provided $16 million for training in substance abuse prevention and CSAT provided $6 million for training in addiction treatment. However, the training focused on service providers, rather than training in research and evaluation (SAMHSA, 1996b). In 1996, SAMHSA developed the Knowledge Development and Application Program (KDA) to develop new

TABLE 2.4 NIDA Funding History (1988–1997): Research Training Grants, Research Grants, and Total Budget (thousands of dollars)

| Year | Research Training Grants | | Research Grants | | Total Budget |
	Amount	Percentage of Total	Amount	Percentage of Total	Amount
1988	$2,298	1.5	$104,658	67.0	$156,252
1989	$2,371	1.0	$165,613	72.6	$228,131
1990	$3,805	1.2	$234,968	71.3	$329,560
1991	$6,808	1.8	$278,727	72.7	$383,656
1992	$7,122	1.8	$289,877	72.6	$399,100
1993	$7,370	1.8	$293,208	72.7	$403,065
1994	$8,325	2.0	$316,665	74.6	$424,315
1995	$9,308	2.1	$329,718	75.5	$436,726
1996	$10,700	2.3	$352,172	76.9	$458,231
1997 (est.)	$11,700	2.4	$377,767	76.3	$494,960

SOURCES: GAO (1994), NIDA (1994), NIH (1997).

TABLE 2.5 NIAAA Funding History (1988–1997): Research Training Grants, Research Grants, and Total Budget (thousands of dollars)

| Year | Research Training Grants | | Research Grants | | Total Budget |
	Amount	Percentage of Total	Amount	Percentage of Total	Amount
1988	$2,590	2.8	$65,454	70.1	$92,763
1989	$2,796	2.3	$88,659	73.9	$120,051
1990	$3,587	2.4	$110,899	74.3	$149,194
1991	$3,548	2.2	$117,647	74.4	$158,141
1992	$3,606	2.1	$128,369	74.9	$171,481
1993	$3,614	2.1	$131,167	74.5	$176,128
1994	$5,029	2.7	$138,180	74.5	$185,538
1995	$5,235	2.7	$142,365	74.7	$190,548
1996	$5,405	2.7	$152,238	76.7	$198,480
1997 (est.)	$5,803	2.7	$164,845	78.0	$211,254

SOURCES: NIAAA (1996) and NIH (1997).

knowledge about ways to improve the prevention and treatment of substance abuse, and to work with state and local governments as well as providers, families, and consumers to apply that knowledge effectively in everyday practice. Outcome measures and evaluation are integral components to each grant program (SAMHSA, 1997).

The private sector devotes even less money than the federal government to any kind of addiction research, training, or treatment development. Although a few foundations support programs related to substance abuse prevention and health services research, most do not. However, a recent survey of foundations did find an encouraging trend; 342 foundations spent a total of $57 million in 1993–1994 to fund prevention programs and media projects (The Foundation Center, 1995). This figure compares favorably with a report which found that during the entire five-year period from 1983 to 1987, 337 foundations awarded a total of $87 million to alcohol and drug abuse programs (The Foundation Center, 1989).

The money spent on research, training, and treatment is, however, a small proportion of the money spent to fight drug abuse and addiction. For example, much of the federal commitment to fight drug addiction is spent on "other related costs" through the Department of Justice, Treasury, Defense, and ONDCP, such as interdiction, intelligence, and incarceration. All of these strategies are important, but there is evidence that treatment is much more cost effective than the kinds of law enforcement efforts that receive most federal funds. According to a RAND study of strategies to decrease drug use, cocaine consumption would be reduced by 1 percent for every $34 million spent on treatment. By contrast, controlling the source of drugs is far more costly; for example, almost $400 million would have to be spent on interdiction to achieve the same 1 percent decrease (RAND, 1994).

The California Drug and Alcohol Treatment Assessment (CALDATA) survey also concluded that treating substance abuse is both effective and cost beneficial indicating a return of $7 for every one dollar invested. Although the cost of treating approximately 150,000 individuals in 1992 totaled more than $200 million, the benefits and returned savings received during treatment and in the year following treatment totaled approximately $1.5 billion. The greatest savings were due mostly to reductions in crime with significant improvements in health and corresponding reductions in hospitalizations (Gerstein et al., 1994).

CONCLUSION

Substance abuse is a prevalent problem affecting millions of Americans. Of particular concern is the growing use of illicit drugs, alcohol, and nicotine by young people. As a result of this growing public health problem, the measurable economic costs of drug addiction clearly are enormous, totaling $257 billion in 1990. However, investments in preventing drug abuse and addiction and in treating addiction appear disproportionately low compared to the resources spent on interdiction and through the criminal justice system—even though there is evidence that treatment is more cost-effective. Resources devoted to research on the causes, prevention, and treatment of addiction are also low compared to the costs of other diseases such as cancer and coronary heart disease. Given the prevalence and cost of addiction, investments in research provide opportunities for understanding the initiation and development of addiction and how addiction can best be prevented and treated, thus, contributing to a decrease in the magnitude of the problem and the cost to society. In order to accomplish this goal, additional resources will be need to attract and train the "best and the brightest" as addiction researchers.

REFERENCES

ACS (American Cancer Society). 1997. *Cancer Facts and Figures, 1997* [http://www.cancer.org/97/facts.html]. March.

AHA (American Heart Association). 1997. *Cardiovascular Disease and Economics* [http//:www.amhrt.org /1997/stats]. March.

Berry RE, Bowland JP. 1977. *The Economic Costs of Alcohol Abuse*. New York: Free Press.

CASA (Center on Addiction and Substance Abuse at Columbia University). 1996. *Substance Abuse and Urban America: Its Impact on an American City, New York.* New York: Center on Addiction and Substance Abuse at Columbia University.

Chen K, Kandel DB. 1995. The natural history of drug use from adolescence to the midthirties in a general population sample. *American Journal of Public Health* 85(1):41–47.

Cruze AM, Harwood JH, Kristiansen PL, Collins JJ, Jones DC. 1981. *Economic Costs to Society of Alcohol and Drug Abuse and Mental Illness, 1977*. Vols. 1 and 2. Report RTI/1923/00-14F. Research Triangle Park, NC: Research Triangle Institute.

Doyle R. 1996. Deaths due to alcohol. *Scientific American* 275(6):30-31. December.

The Foundation Center. 1989. *Alcohol and Drug Abuse Funding: An Analysis of Foundation Grants 1983–1987*. New York: The Foundation Center.

The Foundation Center. 1995. *Grants for Alcohol and Drug Abuse 1995–1996*. New York: The Foundation Center.

GAO (General Accounting Office). 1994. *Drug Abuse Research: Federal Funding and Future Needs*. Gaithersburg, MD: U.S. General Accounting Office.

Gerstein DR, Johnson RA, Harwood HJ, Fountain D, Suter N, Malloy K. 1994. *Evaluating Recovery Services: The California Drug and Alcohol Treatment Assessment (CALDATA)—General Report*. Sacramento, CA: California Department of Drug and Alcohol Programs.

Harwood HJ, Napolitano DM, Kristiansen PL, Collins JJ. 1984. *Economic Costs to Society of Alcohol and Drug Abuse and Mental Illness, 1980*. Report RTI/2734/00-01 FR. Research Triangle Park, NC: Research Triangle Institute.

Institute for Health Policy, Brandeis University. 1993. *Substance Abuse: The Nation's Number One Health Problem, Key Indicators for Policy*. Prepared for the Robert Wood Johnson Foundation, Princeton, NJ. October.

IOM (Institute of Medicine). 1995. *The Development of Medications for the Treatment of Opiate and Cocaine Abuse: Issues for the Government and Private Sector.* Washington, DC: National Academy Press.

IOM. 1996. *Pathways of Addiction.* Washington, DC: National Academy Press.

Johnston LD, O'Malley PM, Bachman JG. 1997. *National Survey Results on Drug Use from the Monitoring the Future Study, 1975–1996.* Ann Arbor, MI: Institute for Social Research, University of Michigan.

Libran CB, Smart RG. 1982. Drinking and drug use among Ontario Indian students. *Drug and Alcohol Dependence* 9:161–171.

May PA. 1989. Alcohol abuse and alcoholism among American Indians: An overview. In: Watts TD, Wright R, eds. *Alcoholism in Minority Populations.* Springfield, IL: Charles C. Thomas. Pp. 95–119.

May PA. 1996. Overview of alcohol abuse epidemiology for American Indian populations. In: Sandefur GD, Rundfuss RR, Cohen B, eds. *Changing Numbers, Changing Needs: American Indian Demography and Public Health.* Washington, DC: National Academy Press. Pp. 235–261.

May PA, Smith MB. 1988. Some Navajo Indian opinions about alcohol abuse and prohibition: A survey and recommendations for policy. *Journal of Studies on Alcohol* 49:324–334.

MMWR (Morbidity and Mortality Weekly Report). 1994. Medical-care expenditures attributable to cigarette smoking—United States, 1993. *Morbidity and Mortality Weekly Report* 43(26):469–472.

MMWR. 1996. Tobacco use and usual source of cigarettes among high school students—United States, 1995. *Morbidity and Mortality Weekly Report* 45(20):413–418.

NCHS (National Center for Health Statistics). 1996. *Health, United States, 1995.* Hyattsville, MD: Public Health Service, U.S. Department of Health and Human Services.

NHLBI (National Heart, Lung, and Blood Institute). 1994. *Morbidity and Mortality: Chartbook on Cardiovascular, Lung, and Blood Diseases.* Washington, DC: National Institutes of Health, Public Health Service, U.S. Department of Health and Human Services.

NIAAA (National Institute on Alcohol Abuse and Alcoholism). 1996. *Research for IOM Committee on Raising the Profile of Drug Abuse and Alcoholism Research.* Rockville, MD: National Institute on Alcohol Abuse and Alcoholism.

NIDA (National Institute on Drug Abuse). 1994. *National Institute on Drug Abuse 1995 Budget Estimate.* Rockville, MD: National Institute on Drug Abuse.

NIH (National Institutes of Health). 1997. Personal communication with Robert Feaga, Office of Financial Management. May 27.

ONDCP (Office of National Drug Control Policy). 1997. *III. Drug Control Funding Tables* [http://www.ncjrs.org/htm/tables.htm]. April 9.

OTA (Office of Technology Assessment). 1985. *Smoking-Related Deaths and Financial Costs.* Washington, DC: OTA Staff Memorandum, Health Program, U.S. Congress.

RAND. 1994. *Controlling Cocaine: Supply Versus Demand Programs.* Santa Monica, CA: RAND Publications.

Rice DP. 1993. The economic cost of alcohol abuse and alcohol dependence: 1990. *Alcohol Health and Research World* 45(1):61–67.

Rice DP. 1995. Personal communication to the Institute of Medicine. University of California at San Francisco. February.

Rice DP, Miller LS. 1996. *Health Economics and Cost Implications of Anxiety and Other Mental Disorders in the United States.* Presented at Satellite Symposium: X World Congress of Psychiatry. Madrid, Spain. August 25. Unpublished.

Rice DP, Hodgson TA, Sinsheimer P, Browner W, Kopstein AN. 1986. The economic costs of the health effects of smoking, 1984. *The Milbank Quarterly* 64(4):489–547.

Rice DP, Kelman S, Dunmeyer S. 1990. *The Economic Costs of Alcohol and Drug Abuse, and Mental Illness: 1985.* DHHS Publication No. (ADM) 90-1694. Washington, DC: Report submitted to the Office of Financing and Coverage Policy of the Alcohol, Drug Abuse, and Mental Health Administration, U.S. Department of Health and Human Services.

Rice DP, Kelman S, Miller LS. 1991a. Economic costs of drug abuse. In: Cartwright WS, Kaple JM, eds. *Economic Costs, Cost-Effectiveness, Financing and Community-Based Drug Treatment.* NIDA Research Monograph 113. Rockville, MD: National Institute on Drug Abuse. Pp. 10–32.

Rice DP, Kelman S, Miller LS. 1991b. Estimates of the economic costs of alcohol and drug abuse and mental illness, 1985 and 1988. *Public Health Reports* 106(3):281–292.

Rice DP, Kelman S, Miller L. 1991c. The economic costs of alcoholism. *Alcohol Health and Research World* 15(4):307–316.

Rice DP, Max W, Novotny T, Shultz J, Hodgson T. 1992. *The Cost of Smoking Revisited: Preliminary Estimates.* Paper presented at the American Public Health Association Annual Meeting. Washington, DC. November 23. Unpublished.

Shultz JM, Novotny TE, Rice DP. 1991a. Quantifying the disease impact of cigarette smoking with SAMMEC II software. *Public Health Reports* 106(3):326–333.

Shultz JM, Rice DP, Parker DL, Goodman RA, Stroh G, Chalmers N. 1991b. Quantifying the disease impact of alcohol use and misuse with ARDI software. *Public Health Reports* 106(4):443–450.

SAMHSA (Substance Abuse and Mental Health Services Administration). 1996a. *Preliminary Estimates from the 1995 National Household Survey on Drug Abuse.* Advance Report No. 18. Rockville, MD: Office of Applied Studies, Substance Abuse and Mental Health Services Administration. August.

SAMHSA. 1996b. Personal communication to the Institute of Medicine. Center for Substance Abuse Prevention. August.

SAMHSA. 1997. *SAMHSA Funding Opportunities* [http://www.samhsa.gov/grant]. March.

Welty TK, Lee ET, Yeh J, Cowan LD, Go O, et al. 1995. Cardiovascular disease risk factors among American Indians: The Strong Heart Study. *American Journal of Epidemiology* 142(3):269–287.

Whittaker JO. 1982. Alcohol and the Standing Rock Sioux Tribe: A twenty-year follow-up study. *Journal of Studies on Alcohol* 43:191–200.

Winfree LT, Griffiths CT. 1985. Trends in drug orientations and behavior: Changes in a rural community, 1975–1982. *International Journal of the Addictions* 20(10):1495–1508.

Winfree LT, Griffiths CT, Sellers CS. 1989. Social learning theory, drug use, and American Indian youths: A cross-cultural test. *Justice Quarterly* 6(3):395–417.

Varmus H. 1995. *Disease-Specific Estimates of Direct and Indirect Costs of Illness and NIH Support.* Bethesda, MD: Office of the Director, National Institutes of Health, Public Health Service, U.S. Department of Health and Human Services.

3

Neurobiology of Addiction: An Overview

This chapter presents a brief overview of the underlying neurobiology of drug addiction and suggests a perspective with which to put the neurobiological findings in context with the social, psychological, and environmental aspects of drug addiction. The chapter is not intended to be a comprehensive review of these topics. Rather, its intent is to demonstrate for new investigators, students, university administrators, and policymakers the richness of basic research regarding abuse of alcohol and other drugs and to provide the lay reader with a greater understanding of the role of the brain in the transition from drug use to addiction. Some of the key advances in research into the neurobiology of addiction are also summarized in Appendix F.

The role of dopamine as a neurotransmitter in the brain reward circuitry is highlighted in this chapter, because it relates to the four classes of drugs discussed in this report—nicotine, alcohol, stimulants, and opioids. Although there are some important differences among them, these drugs share common reward pathways in the brain. Fundamental neurobiological research as outlined in this chapter, together with findings from clinical and behavioral and social science research (see Chapter 4), are providing researchers with neurobiological answers that offer better ways to understand, prevent, or treat drug addiction.

At the heart of our current understanding of addiction is the idea that in vulnerable individuals, the disease of addiction is produced by the interaction of the drugs themselves with genetic, environmental, psychosocial, behavioral, and other factors, which causes long-lived alterations in the biochemical and functional properties of selected groups of neurons in the brain. In particular, addictive drugs, when taken with adequate dose, frequency, and chronicity, appear to commandeer circuits intimately involved in the control of emotion and motivation, thus impairing the insight and volitional control of the addicted person. At the same time, the alterations produced by chronic drug use facilitate the formation of deeply ingrained emotional memories that predispose to drug craving and hence to relapse.

Thus, in developing a conceptual understanding of addiction, it must be acknowledged that compulsive drug use cannot be understood from any single level of analysis. The development of drug addiction, at a minimum, involves the properties of the drugs involved, the neural circuits on which they operate,

---

BOX 3.1
Animal Models: Examples from Alcohol Research

Experimental laboratory animal models remain an essential resource in modern biomedical research because large segments of investigation require the intact animal. This is particularly true for behavioral disorders, including the addictive disorders, and self-administration models are particularly useful for studying all psychoactive substances in animals. Self-administration models, although they vary in specific aspects, all involve making the animals capable of administering drugs to themselves by performing some action, such as pressing a bar or entering a chamber.

Consistent self-administration of alcohol can be established in primates, rodents, and other animals. These techniques have contributed to better understanding of the behavioral and biological conditions of ethanol intake. In many aspects, these procedures mimic the "learning to drink" phenomenon evident in humans. These procedures are used to study the pharmacodynamic effects of ethanol, such as acute intoxication, tolerance, and dependence, and to study the medical consequences of chronic ingestion; for example, fetal alcohol syndrome (FAS), brain damage, and liver disease. Self-administration models are particularly useful in studying the behavioral patterns and consequences of ethanol ingestion.

The finding that food deprivation leads to increased ethanol intake in ethanol self-administration models provides a better understanding of the relationship between drug use and eating disorders. Alcohol is also commonly taken with other drugs and the self-administration model, where animals, like humans, take in substantial quantities of drugs and become dependent, also provides a means to examine the outcomes of multiple drug use. Further, animal self-administration models provide opportunities to examine the effects of potential medications for the treatment of alcohol dependence (e.g., naltrexone). Test medications are also evaluated to determine whether they sustain drug taking or might be abused. The strength of this model is such that the Food and Drug Administration (FDA) and Drug Enforcement Administration (DEA) rely heavily on self-administration evaluations to determine the "abuse liability" of drugs for purposes of scheduling under the Controlled Substances Act.

an individual's genetic makeup and developmental experiences, the presence or absence of psychological distress or psychiatric illness, and the sociocultural context in which drugs might be used. A sophisticated understanding of how the brain works recognizes that an individual's life experience and social context exert powerful effects on the brain and, therefore, on behavior.

THE BRAIN'S COMMON "REWARD" PATHWAY

Two lines of investigation led to the conclusion that addictive drugs, although chemically different from one another, all affect a brain system involved in the control of motivated behavior. The first set of experiments were performed in rats in the 1950s and involved stimulating discrete brain regions (Olds and Milner, 1954). In these experiments, the discovery was made that there were a small number of brain regions in which stimulation was "pleasurable" or "rewarding" because the rats would press a lever tens of thousands of times in succession, ignoring normal needs for food, water, and rest, to gain electrical stimulation (self-stimulation; see also Box 3.1). In the popular literature these regions were called "the pleasure center" but scientifically they are better described as "brain reward regions" (i.e., regions in which electrical activation profoundly reinforces the lever-pressing behavior) (Wise, 1978).

A great deal of research since the 1950s has established that the major brain circuit mediating this type of reinforcement is a pathway extending from the ventral tegmental area (VTA), an area within the midbrain (a part of the brainstem), to a structure called the nucleus accumbens (NAc) (Figure 3.1). The NAc is particularly interesting because it occupies the crossroads between a group of brain structures, called the limbic system, that are primarily involved in the control of emotion, and another part of the brain, the striatum, that is involved in the initiation and control of movement. Nerve cells (neurons) in the brain communicate with each other using diverse chemical substances called neurotransmitters. One of the major neurotransmitters used in the brain reward circuit is dopamine (Wise, 1978).

The depiction of the interaction of a nerve cell (neuron) in the VTA with a neuron in the NAc (Figure 3.1) represents a general model of neuronal communication. Neurons communicate using chemical neurotransmitters such as dopamine—one of more than 100 chemical substances that are used for cell-to-cell communication in the nervous system. The neurotransmitter is stored in the transmitting neuron and released when the neuron is stimulated. The transmitter diffuses across a specialized divide called a synapse and binds to receptors, which are specialized recognition sites. Depending on the transmitter, the receiving or "postsynaptic" neurons will be excited or inhibited, or will undergo more complex biochemical alterations (Cooper et al., 1996).

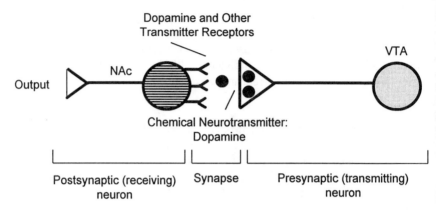

FIGURE 3.1 Schematic diagram of the brain reward circuitry. NOTE: NAc = nucleus accumbens; VTA = ventral tegmental area.

The second set of clues concerning the substrates of addiction came from more recent work which showed that each of these highly addictive drugs mimics or enhances the actions of one or more neurotransmitters in the brain that are involved in the control of the brain reward circuit (Cooper et al., 1996). The opioids mimic endogenous opioid-like compounds called endorphins; cocaine and related drugs enhance the actions of dopamine itself; nicotine mimics the action of acetylcholine (another transmitter) at its nicotinic receptors; and alcohol, among its many effects, facilitates the activation of a particular receptor for gamma-aminobutyric acid (GABA), one of the most prevalent neurotransmitters throughout the brain. Although each of these four mimicked neurotransmitters has many actions in the brain, they all share one common property: all regulate the activity of the brain reward pathway that extends from the VTA to the NAc (Di Chiara and Imperato, 1988).

Each of these abused drugs also interacts with other neurotransmitter systems and molecules within neurons that act as "second messengers" that effectively translate input to neurons into a variety of intracellular chemical and molecular changes (signal transduction), some of which affect gene expression. In addition, other types of neurotransmitters can be affected in direct and indirect ways. For example, one way neurons regulate the amount of neurotransmitter acting at a second neuron is through reuptake mechanisms, that is, the reabsorption of the transmitter into the presynaptic neuron via specialized channels called "transporters." Cocaine inhibits the neuronal reuptake of serotonin and norepinephrine, as well as dopamine, leaving these neurotransmitters in the synapse and effectively increasing their actions within the synapse by increasing their action on their receptors. These additional actions contribute to the unique properties of each class of abused agents and may enhance or reduce the behavioral reinforcement associated with activation of dopamine pathways (Koob, 1996).

As described, the major neurotransmitter released by VTA neurons in the NAc is dopamine. Experiments in which dopamine neurons are destroyed, or other experiments in which dopamine receptors are blocked, confirm that this neurotransmitter is necessary for significant brain reward. Cocaine and the related synthetic compound, amphetamine, both facilitate the action of dopamine while also affecting the balance of other neurotransmitters.

DRUG EFFECTS ON BRAIN REWARD SYSTEMS

Normally, following the release of dopamine, its action is terminated by a presynaptic reuptake transporter that takes the dopamine back into the neuron that released it (the presynaptic neuron). **Cocaine** mimics dopamine enough to bind to the dopamine reuptake transporter, but not enough to be taken up. Hence, cocaine blocks the transporter, causing a buildup of dopamine in the synapse because it is not inactivated by reuptake. **Amphetamine** causes the presynaptic neuron to release more dopamine, essentially by putting the transporter into "reverse." Thus, both cocaine and amphetamine produce strong stimulation of the dopamine pathway leading to the brain reward centers (Hyman, 1996) (Figure 3.2).

Opioids are hypothesized to act on the brain reward circuitry in at least two ways. There are opioid receptors on neurons in the limbic system, including the NAc; thus opioids may act on these brain regions directly. In addition, opioids can indirectly cause VTA neurons to release more dopamine. The firing rate of VTA dopamine neurons is held at a certain "tonic" or stable level by inhibitory neurons. These inhibitory neurons, in turn, possess opioid receptors. Because opioids are inhibitory, endogenous opioids (e.g., enkephalins) or opioid drugs (e.g., morphine) essentially turn off or decrease the action of these inhibitory neurons (Nicoll et al., 1980) and thereby disinhibit the midbrain dopamine neurons. This results in enhanced release of dopamine and a stronger stimulation of the brain reward centers and imbalance with other neurotransmitters (Johnson and North, 1992; Izenwasser et al., 1993).

Although less well understood, both *alcohol* (ethanol) (Tabakoff and Hoffman, 1996) and *nicotine* (Dani and Heinemann, 1996) appear to disinhibit VTA neurons and to cause dopamine release in this same circuit. Ethanol increases the firing of dopamine neurons in the ventral tegmental area (VTA) and increases extracellular dopamine levels in the nucleus accumbens (NAc). The sites at which ethanol exerts it action may be multiple and include a number of modulators of dopaminergic activity in the VTA and the NAc (See Box 3.2). These (and other) neurotransmitter systems and sites may also be involved in mediating negative reinforcement by ethanol, as with drinking for relief of withdrawal symptoms and anxiety (Koob, 1992a).

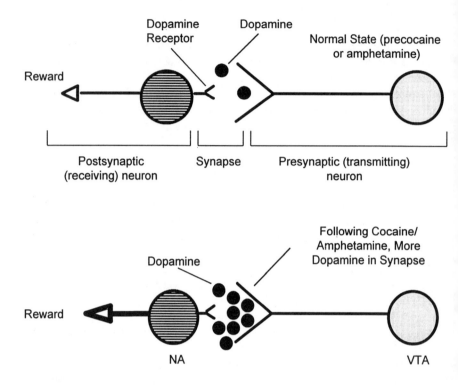

FIGURE 3.2 The effect of cocaine and amphetamine. NOTE: NAc = nucleus accumbens; VTA = ventral tegmental area.

EMOTION, MEMORY, AND THE TRANSITION
FROM USE TO ADDICTION

In addition to the reward pathways, the human brain contains multiple circuits that are involved in the processing of emotion, learning, and conditioning. These "emotional circuits" are adaptive survival circuits; they assign significance (e.g., dangerous, edible, desirable) to individuals, things, and events in the world, and then regulate the functioning of both the input and output circuits of the brain to produce adaptive responses, including escape, approach, and aggression. Connections between brain circuits mediating emotional states and those that mediate the encoding of memories underlie the development of memories with strong or weak emotional components. If strong enough, such memory can be quite simple, as when a child burns his or her finger, and a single experience will dominate subsequent behavior. However, most memories are complex and involve multiple emotional components.

BOX 3.2
Effects of Alcohol on Neurotransmission

Ethanol differs from other psychotropic drugs in that it produces primary-level effects on multiple receptor systems, ion channels, and signal trans-duction pathways both in the brain and in peripheral organ systems. Recent evidence has shown that ethanol potentiation of the GABA$_A$ receptor requires phosporylation of the gamma 2L splice variant of the GABA$_A$ receptor by the gamma isoform of protein kinase C (PKC) (Harris et al., 1995; Wafford and Whiting, 1992; Wafford et al., 1991). Mutant knockout mice without the PKC$_\gamma$ isozyme lack ethanol responsive actions on cerebellar membrane prepara-tions and show reduced behavioral and physiological responses to alcohol while retaining sensitivity to barbiturate and benzodiazepine drugs (Harris et al., 1995). However, alcohol also affects the functioning of other systems in a less direct way, which results in an enhancement or decrease in the activity of many other neurotransmitters, ions, enzymes, and other cellular proc-esses in the brain and elsewhere. Because it is freely permeable across cell membranes, ethanol also disrupts intracellular metabolic processes and sig-nal transduction pathways in neuronal cells as well as cells in other organs (e.g., liver, heart, pancreas) (Li, 1983). Studies in the last 15 years have shown that ethanol (in concentrations that produce behavioral effects) affects the function of several membrane receptors which regulate the flow of ions through other membrane molecules that serve as ion channels (ligand-gated ion channels). In this way, ethanol causes an increase in the flow of chloride ions mediated by a specific type of GABA receptor (the GABA$_A$-benzodiazepine receptor complex) and decreases calcium ion flow mediated by other receptor types (the NMDA-glutamate receptor system). Ethanol also affects a specific type of serotonin receptor that mediates ion channel func-tion to enhance the flow of sodium and potassium ions. Cell-to-cell differ-ences as well as regional differences in sensitivity of these ligand-gated ion channels to ethanol have been discovered. Such differences help explain some of the varied behavioral effects produced by ethanol, for example, re-lease of inhibition, sedation, and memory impairment. Chronically, ethanol causes long-term neuroadaptive changes in the function of the GABA$_A$-benzodiazepine receptor complex and the NMDA-glutamate receptor com-plex, which contribute to the production of chronic tolerance.

A second group of signal transduction pathways that ethanol affects are the G-protein coupled and adenylate cyclase related receptors, whose acti-vating ligands include the opioid peptides, dopamine, serotonin, and adeno-sine. Chronically, ethanol, through actions on G proteins, causes changes in the activity of neurons in pathways mediated by the opioid peptides, sero-tonin, and dopamine, which also contribute to the development of tolerance (Fitzgerald and Nestler, 1995).

The dopaminergic pathway that extends from the VTA to the NAc is part of an emotional circuit that likely evolved to motivate behaviors required for survival and reproductive success, such as sexual behaviors. When something is highly rewarding, memories of that experience are likely to be vivid, complete with positive emotional overtones, and a remembrance of the circumstances under which it was encountered. Thus, the dopaminergic reward pathway likely plays a role in assigning novel stimuli to specific adaptive behavioral repertoires. By perverse serendipity, this adaptive emotional circuit makes brains vulnerable to drug addiction because certain addictive drugs mimic or enhance the actions of neurotransmitters used within it. Thus, drugs of abuse and addiction tap into and "short circuit" powerful emotional circuitry in the brain (Koob, 1996). An important implication is that drug addiction research may be one of the most promising windows on the neurobiology of emotions elicited by nondrug stimuli. Indeed, addictive drugs provide very important information about how the brain normally functions.

All addictive drugs have actions outside the dopaminergic brain reward circuit as well as within it. The sum total of a drug's actions in the brain is determined by where receptors for that drug are found, and what those receptors do. Because all addictive drugs have both a common site of action—the brain reward pathway—and unshared sites of action, their subjective and objective behavioral properties differ. Thus, for example, both cocaine and opioids are reinforcing, but opioids are sedating, while cocaine is a powerful stimulant (O'Brien, 1996).

Some of the actions of cocaine depend on interactions with serotonergic systems. Cocaine increases extracellular serotonin levels by inhibiting the reuptake of previously released serotonin in much the same way that it inhibits the reuptake of dopamine. There is a diffuse network of serotonin-releasing neurons projecting to the VTA and NAc (Phelix and Broderick, 1995); activation of this system probably facilitates dopamine release in the NAc. The activity of the VTA to NAc neurons that appear to be so important in reward processes are also subject to regulation by several neuropeptides, including the endogenous opioids (as discussed above) and two other brain peptides that function as neuromodulators, cholecystokinin-8 (CCK-8) (Hamilton and Freeman, 1995) and neurotensin (Steinberg et al., 1995). Treatments that affect the release or actions of these neuropeptides may also alter the functions of reward pathways.

The neural locations of the receptors or transporters through which drugs act are obviously of primary importance in determining their effects, but other properties of a drug also appear to be important determinants of the abuse potential of drugs. Drugs are most reinforcing when their level in the brain rises very rapidly. Thus, drugs that are smoked or injected produce far more powerful effects than drugs taken orally, in part because they reach the brain so rapidly when administered in this way. Yet, it is clear, and well represented by the case of alcohol, that orally delivered drugs also can produce profound effects and dependence. It is an obvious but important point that purer or more potent forms of drugs also have more powerful effects on the brain. Purity and route of administration explain why smoked cocaine free base (e.g., "crack" cocaine, which when smoked, produces volatilized pure drug exposed to the lungs' massive surface area) is far more quickly addictive than powdered cocaine hydrochloride absorbed via the nasal mucosa, which is, in turn, far more quickly addictive than chewed coca leaves, where the cocaine is absorbed more slowly from the mouth and gastrointestinal tract (and partially destroyed by digestive enzymes) (Wilkinson et al., 1980). The form in which a drug is used, however, may also create barriers to use. For example, smoking is not initially natural and may cause coughing and other discomfort. Thus a certain amount of social pressure or support for smoking is needed to get young people over this initial barrier before they find tobacco smoking pleasurable and put themselves at risk for addiction. Taking alcohol or other drugs orally in liquid or tablet form does not present this type of barrier, so initial use may be easier to achieve.

People report that they take drugs to gain pleasure, to produce alterations in consciousness, to conform to the behavior of their peers, and to relieve stress and other negative emotions. However, the fact that certain drugs produce subjective euphoria or relieve dysphoria in humans and are reinforcing in animal models does not necessarily mean that they will produce addiction (i.e., inability to control use despite serious negative consequences; see Chapter 1). Indeed, over time, the addicted person's enjoyment of drug-taking is decreased because tolerance develops or medical complications ensue. Despite diminished enjoyment, the life of the addicted person revolves around the obtaining, using, and recovering from the effects of the drug despite problems at home and work and failure in life roles. The effects of the drug and circumstances of use are somehow so important that the addicted individual may go to great lengths to deny that its use is causing any difficulty. The denial, manipulation, and dishonesty that the addicted person frequently exhibits in the service of ongoing drug use may frustrate and anger family members, colleagues, and caregivers.

A key point in our current understanding of the neurobiology of drug abuse is that there is good evidence that use of a drug at an adequate dose with adequate frequency and chronicity produces long-lived changes in brain functioning. Many of these changes represent compensatory adaptations (homeostatic responses) to excessive bombardment by the drug. It is these drug-induced changes in brain function that produce addiction in some individuals.

The types of long-term changes that addictive drugs produce in the brain now can be divided conceptually into three categories. First, opioids and ethyl alcohol, but not cocaine, produce compensatory adaptations in brain regions that control somatic functions, thus producing physical dependence. As a result, discontinuation of opioids or alcohol can produce a physical withdrawal syndrome, such as the well-known alcohol withdrawal syndrome that includes hypertension, rapid heartbeat, tremor, nystagmus, insomnia, and grand mal seizures (O'Brien, 1996).

Second, all addictive drugs appear to produce adaptations within the brain reward circuitry itself. These are quite complex and far from fully understood. A subset of these adaptations contributes to tolerance, decreasing some of the reinforcing effects of the drug and therefore contributing to increases in the dosage needed to achieve a desired level of effect. The same types of adaptations that contribute to tolerance also contribute to dependence, that is, putting the brain in a state that will lead to emotional and motivational symptoms of withdrawal (e.g., depressed mood, inability to experience pleasure, and drug craving) following drug cessation. At the same time there is evidence for other types of adaptations in brain reward circuits that may produce sensitization (i.e., the concept that some drug effects may actually get stronger with repeated stimulation). Some aspects of sensitization increase craving for the drug; others, like the syndrome of cocaine-induced paranoia that may develop with chronic use, create novel difficulties for drug users (Satel et al., 1991).

A third category of long-term alteration in brain function that may be produced by addictive drugs in some individuals is the production of powerful "emotional memories" of drug use. There is increasing evidence to suggest that things learned in the context of strong emotional activation are most indelibly etched into distinct memories. Among the most dramatic examples of this phenomenon are seen in individuals suffering from posttraumatic stress disorder (PTSD); for a PTSD survivor, even minor cues can bring the entire traumatic episode flooding back into consciousness, including the related emotions. The dopaminergic circuitry activated by drugs of abuse may be directly involved in setting the strength of memories associated with reinforcement. Thus, places, persons, and bodily feelings that have been connected with drug use may be stored in memory in such a way that cues recalling drug experiences may elicit strong drug cravings (O'Brien, 1976; Wilker, 1973). Well-known examples include the craving for a cigarette produced by a large meal or the reexperiencing of some withdrawal symptoms by detoxified heroin addicts who return to a site at which they had previously used drugs. The relationship of these cue-dependent memories to relapse in previously detoxified individuals is currently a matter of study (IOM, 1996). In addition, behavioral therapies (e.g., cognitive-behavioral psychotherapy, supportive-expressive psychotherapy, interpersonal psychotherapy, 12-step facilitation, and motivational enhancement therapy; also see Chapter 4) have been developed to help detoxified individuals cope with circumstances that elicit craving (Beck et al., 1990; Carroll et al., 1991; Luborsky et al., 1995; Marlatt and Gordon, 1985; NIAAA, 1994a,b, 1995; Prochaska and DiClemente, 1986).

These different types of long-term changes in the brain have varied time courses of onset and decay. Somatic withdrawal may last from days to one or two weeks; the motivational aspects of withdrawal may last from several weeks to months; emotional memories related to drug use may last a lifetime. Drug abuse researchers are now beginning to uncover many of the details of the mechanisms by which drugs alter the functioning of the brain.

VULNERABILITIES TO ADDICTION

In this brief chapter it is not possible to address all the reasons why some individuals who use addictive drugs become dependent and others do not, and why some stop using and others do not. Risk factors for becoming addicted are as yet poorly understood but can be divided into factors that increase consumption and factors that increase the likelihood that the individual will be captured by the drug. Both genetic and environmental factors likely influence both the willingness of an individual to experiment with drugs and alcohol as well as the risk of developing dependence.

There is very little known currently about potential genetic contributions to vulnerability to opiate, cocaine, or nicotine addiction. However, most researchers agree, based on three types of investigations, that there are clear genetic components to vulnerability to alcoholism. These investigations are twin and adoption studies, genetic studies of certain human populations, and animal studies. Twin and adoption studies have demonstrated that early onset alcoholism is strongly influenced in males and females by genetic factors. Later onset alcoholism seems less influenced by genetic factors and more strongly influenced by environmental and emotional factors (Cloninger et al., 1989; Heath et al., 1991a,b; Kendler et al., 1992).

Genetic studies have focused on individuals in populations in which many people exhibit a strong aversive physiological reaction to alcohol (alcohol flush reaction), which is sometimes inaccurately called an allergy to alcohol. It includes facial flushing, rapid heartbeat, and headaches. The alcohol flush reaction, which if severe enough can cause loss of consciousness, occurs in roughly half of people with Chinese and Japanese ancestry and about a third of people with Korean ancestry. The flush reaction may represent a physiological "protective" factor that tends to prevent affected individuals from developing an alcohol addiction. The biological basis of this flush reaction is a variation in two genes that code for two principal enzymes of alcohol metabolism, alcohol dehydrogenase (ADH) and an aldehyde dehydrogenase (ALDH2) located in a specific part of cells called mitochondria (Thomasson et al., 1991). The most alcohol-sensitive individuals in these populations are those who inherit from both parents (homozygous) the gene variant that causes ALDH2 deficiency; these individuals cannot drink even small amounts of alcohol. If only one such gene is inherited (heterozygous), the individual can drink but is less able to drink large quantities and is 4-6 times less likely to become addicted. Individuals with the variant gene for ADH are also less likely to become addicted, but the effect is not as great. Interestingly, Caucasians, Alaskan Natives, and Native American populations exhibit very low prevalence rates for these genetic variations (Thomasson et al., 1994).

Genetic vulnerability to alcohol addiction can also be studied in animal models, including rats, mice, and even fruit flies (see Appendix D). Several rat strains have been developed through selective breeding that exhibit high or low alcohol preference in self-administration models (Li et al., 1993). These animal models have characteristics that mirror in many respects human alcohol addiction; the animals show tolerance development, and pharmacological agents (e.g., naltrexone, an opiate antagonist) that reduce alcohol consumption in humans also reduce consumption in the animals (Li and McBride, 1995; Schuckit, 1994). Inbred and recombinant strains of mice have also been developed to assess the contributions of multiple genes to alcohol- (and drug-) related responses. Using a method called quantitative trait loci gene mapping (QTL), specific parts of genes have been identified that are associated with a variety of alcohol-related traits, including alcohol preference, sensitivity, tolerance, and withdrawal (Crabbe et al., 1994).

The search for specific genes that may confer enhanced risk of alcoholism has already progressed significantly, and much interest is focused on variant genes that may increase vulnerability to other types of addiction. The study of environmental factors that produce risk versus resilience with respect to drug addiction, however, must contend with multiple behavioral, psychological, and social factors that complicate analysis. In addition, other factors influence drug taking, including drug availability, acceptability in the individual's subculture, behavioral alternatives to drug use, and presence of other psychiatric illness. Factors that influence the "capture rate" include the intrinsic addictiveness of the drug used and, as mentioned above, the form in which it is administered (e.g., smoked crack cocaine).

In the model that has been outlined here, addiction is a disease of the nervous system, interacting with other biological systems and behavioral and environmental factors, that markedly impairs a person's ability to control his or her drug-seeking behavior; in fact, it makes resumption of drinking or drug-taking a compelling risk for the individual despite the highly negative effects of drug addiction on the individual's health and well-being.

Without building a greater context, however, such a biological model could contribute to the common misconception that if alcoholism or drug addiction is not simply willful misbehavior, addicted individuals cannot be held responsible for their actions. Individuals predisposed to developing coronary artery disease, for example, are not castigated by their physicians, but they are asked to follow a certain diet, to exercise, and to comply with medication regimens. Yet, for many individuals, the behavioral changes required to cope with heart disease are difficult and relapses to well-ingrained patterns are common. The same concept should be applied by physicians and society to those addicted to alcohol, nicotine, or illicit drugs. As in the treatment of heart disease, the best therapeutic results are obtained when addicted persons are given responsibility for themselves once a diagnosis is made and treatment recommended.

The clinically critical difference between addiction and coronary artery disease, however, is that the disease of addiction markedly diminishes the ability of the patient to follow through on medical advice. Hard as it is for patients with coronary artery disease to comply with treatment it is even harder for addicted patients to comply. Thus, much research is devoted to finding medications to treat drug addiction (e.g., methadone) or to reduce drug cravings (e.g., naltrexone) (IOM, 1995). In addition, the clinician, as well as the patient's family, friends, and employers, must serve as a bulwark for the patient, against the intense drive for another drink, one more cigarette, or a few puffs of crack cocaine.

The idea that addictive drugs may commandeer key motivational circuits in the brain should also help researchers, physicians, and others to understand some of the otherwise inexplicable behavior of addicted people, who continue to use drugs either openly or surreptitiously despite, in many cases, tremendously negative personal and social consequences. This model also implies the importance of prevention and underlines the fact that, for those who are most severely affected, recovery may never be complete when environmental cues can always engender intense cravings and risk of relapse.

CONCLUSION

Recent discoveries have turned addiction research into a mature field that should attract the very best scientists interested in both basic and translational research. Researchers have cloned the brain receptors (i.e., the immediate molecular targets) for all significant drugs of abuse and have defined their locations in the brain. Of great significance, there is now general agreement on the importance of the dopaminergic brain reward pathway as one of the key common sites of action of addictive drugs. For example, because of the positive correlation between the potencies of cocaine as dopamine reuptake blockers and their ability to maintain self-administration behavior, it has been suggested that the action of cocaine at its binding site mediates the effects that contribute to abuse (Fischman and Johanson, 1996; Bergman et al., 1989; Ritz et al., 1987). Opioids and nicotine also stimulate the release of dopamine triggering the dopaminergic brain reward pathway (Corrigall et al., 1992; Koob, 1992b). Some aspects of treatment for all drugs are beginning to capitalize on the identification of this common pathway and the systems that regulate it. For example, naltrexone, an orally effective and long-acting opioid antagonist, has been shown effective in preventing relapse to opiate dependence in extremely motivated people (i.e., under strong external pressure to remain opiate free) (Brahen et al., 1978). Naltrexone has been shown to be effective in reducing relapse to alcohol dependence (O'Malley et al., 1996; Volpicelli et al., 1992). Nalmefene, a newer opioid antagonist, is currently undergoing testing and appears to have positive effects similar to those of naltrexone (Mason et al., 1994).

Researchers can now turn to the very difficult problems of understanding the precise brain mechanisms by which drugs alter brain function and come to dominate behavior. Table 3.1 lists some of these compelling research questions for the future. In the process, a great deal will be learned about the normal control of motivation and emotion in the brain. With such discoveries, understanding about other human diseases and illnesses can also increase. For example, dopamine systems are not only the substrates of drug abuse and addiction, but also of psychotic symptoms that occur in a variety of psychiatric disorders and of some movement disorders, such as Parkinson's disease.

The importance of these areas and findings notwithstanding, it must be emphasized that drug addiction is the result of interacting biological, behavioral, social, and environmental factors. Thus successful treatment can come only from integrative research efforts involving multiple disciplines.

TABLE 3.1 Some Future Challenges in Basic Research

- Identification of factors leading to susceptibility or resistance to drug abuse in animals
- Analysis of the inputs to and outputs from brain reward pathways: How does stimulation of these pathways produce reinforcement?
- Development of better animal models, suitable for simultaneous genetic analysis, genetic manipulation, and behavioral analysis
- Development of targeted, conditional gene knockout technologies and continued development of conditional gene activation technologies in transgenic animals (both are broad needs in neuroscience)
- Dopamine: identification of which of the five distinct dopamine receptors are involved in mediating reward responses
- Animal models: production of genetically engineered animals in which the genes for individual dopamine receptors or the dopamine transporter can be selectively inactivated in an inducible fashion; assess susceptibility of animals to drug consumption and drug addiction before and after genetic manipulations
- Determination of the neurobiological basis of nicotine reinforcement
- Molecular studies identifying genes, posttranslational modifications, or signal transduction pathways that produce functional subtypes of mu, kappa, and delta opioid receptors
- Development of selective agonists or antagonists of kappa and delta opioid receptors for use in humans
- Further characterization and evaluation of vaccine approaches to cocaine addiction
- Identification of genes and quantitative tract loci associated with alcohol-related phenotypes in animal models
- Elucidation of neurobiology and molecular biology underlying alcohol tolerance
- Use of transgenic and gene knockout animal models to evaluate alcohol responses on brain neurotransmitter and reward systems
- Evaluation of the role of N-methyl-D-aspartate and nitric oxide pathways on alcohol neurotoxicity, tolerance, and cognitive impairment
- Elucidation of neuropeptide effects (e.g., corticotropin-releasing factor [CRF], neurotensin, arginine vasopressin [AVP]) and neurosteroid effects on alcohol actions and alcohol withdrawal

REFERENCES

Beck AT, Wright FD, Newman CF. 1990. *Cognitive Therapy of Cocaine Abuse.* Philadelphia: Center for Cognitive Therapy.

Bergman J, Madras BK, Johnson SE, Spealman RD. 1989. Effects of cocaine and related drugs in nonhuman primates. Part III. Self-administration by squirrel monkeys. *Journal of Pharmacology and Experimental Therapeutics* 251:150–155.

Brahen LS, Capone T, Bloom S, et al. 1978. An alternative to methadone for probationer addicts: Narcotic antagonist treatment. *Contemporary Drug Issues* 13:117–132.

Carroll ME, Carmona GG, May SA. 1991. V. Cocaine self-administration in rats: Effects of non-drug alternative reinforcers on acquisition. *Psychopharmacology* 110:5–12.

Cloninger CR, Sigvardsson S, Gilligan SB, Von Knorring AL, Reich T, Bohman M. 1989. Genetic heterogeneity and the classification of alcoholism. *Advances in Alcoholism and Substance Abuse* 7(3/4):3–16.

Cooper JR, Bloom FE, Roth RH. 1996. Cellular foundation of neuropharmacology. In: *The Biochemical Basis of Neuropharmacology.* 7th Edition. New York: Oxford University Press. Pp. 9–48.

Corrigall WA, Franklin KBJ, Coen KM, Clarke PBS. 1992. The mesolimbic dopamine system is implicated in the reinforcing effects of nicotine. *Psychopharmacology (Berl)* 107:285–289.

Crabbe JC, Belknap JK, Buck KJ. 1994. Genetic animal models of alcohol and drug abuse. *Science* 264:1715–1723.

Dani JA, Heinemann S. 1996. Molecular and cellular aspects of nicotine abuse. *Neuron* 16:905–908.

Di Chiara G, Imperato A. 1988. Drugs abused by humans preferentially increase synaptic dopamine concentrations in the mesolimbic system of freely moving rats. *Proceedings of the National Academy of Sciences of the United States of America* 85:5274–5278.

Fischman MW, Johanson CE. 1996. Cocaine. In: Schuster CR, Gust SW, Kuhar MJ, eds. *Pharmacological Aspects of Drug Dependence: Towards an Integrated Neurobehavioral Approach. Handbook of Experimental Pharmacology* 118:159–195.

Fitzgerald LW, Nestler EJ. 1995. Molecular and cellular adaptations in signal transduction pathways following ethanol exposure. *Clinical Neuroscience* 3:165–173.

Hamilton ME, Freeman AS. 1995. Effects of administration of cholecystokinin into the VTA on DA overflow in nucleus accumbens and amygdala of freely moving rats. *Brain Research* 688:134–142.

Harris RA, McQuilkin SJ, Paylor R, Abeliovich A, Tonegawa S, Wehner JM. 1995. Mutant mice lacking the gamma-isoform of protein kinase C show decreased behavioral actions of ethanol and altered function of gamma-aminobutyrate type A receptors. *Proceedings of the National Academy of Sciences of the United States of America* 92(9):3658–3662.

Heath AC, Meyer J, Eaves LJ, Martin NG. 1991a. The inheritance of alcohol consumption patterns in a general population twin sample: I. Multidimensional scaling of quantity/frequency data. *Journal of Studies on Alcohol* 52(4):345–352.

Heath AC, Meyer J, Jardine R Martin NG. 1991b. The inheritance of alcohol consumption patterns in a general population twin sample: II. Determinants of consumption frequency and quantity consumed. *Journal of Studies on Alcohol* 52(5):425–433.

Hyman SE. 1996. Addiction to cocaine and amphetamine. *Neuron* 16:901–904.

IOM (Institute of Medicine). 1995. *The Development of Medications for the Treatment of Opiate and Cocaine Addictions.* Washington, D.C.: National Academy Press.

IOM. 1996. *Pathways of Addiction: Opportunities in Drug Abuse Research.* Washington, D.C.: National Academy Press.

Izenwasser S, Búzás B, Cox BM. 1993. Differential regulation of adenylyl cyclase activity by mu- and delta-opioids in rat caudate-putamen and nucleus accumbens. *Journal of Pharmacology and Experimental Therapeutics* 267:145–152.

Johnson SW, North RA. 1992. Opioids excite dopamine neurons by hyperpolarization of local interneurons. *Journal of Neuroscience* 12:483–488.

Kendler KS, Heath AC, Neale MC, Kessler RC, Eaves LJ. 1992. A population-based twin study of alcoholism in women. *Journal of the American Medical Association* 268(14):1877–1882.

Koob GF. 1992a. Drugs of abuse: Anatomy, pharmacology, and function of reward pathways. *Trends in Pharmacological Sciences* 13:177–184.

Koob GF. 1992b. Dopamine, addiction and reward. *Seminars in the Neurosciences* 4:139–148.

Koob GF. 1996. Drug addiction: The yin and yang of hedonistic homeostasis. *Neuron* 16:893–896.

Li T-K. 1983. The absorption, distribution and metabolism of ethanol and its effects on nutrition and hepatic function. In: Tabakoff B, Sutker PB, Randall CL, eds. *Medical and Social Aspects of Alcohol Abuse.* New York: Plenum Publishing. Pp. 44–77.

Li T-K, McBride WJ. 1995. Pharmacogenetic models of alcoholism. *Clinical Neuroscience* 3:182–188.

Li T-K, Lumeng L, Doolittle DP. 1993. Selective breeding for alcohol preference and associated responses. *Behavior Genetics* 23:163–170.

Luborsky L, Woody GE, Hole A, Velleco A. 1995. Supportive-expressive dynamic psychotherapy for treatment of opiate drug dependence. In: Barber JP, Crits-Christoph P, eds. *Dynamic Therapies for Psychiatric Disorders (Axis I).* New York: Basic Books. Pp. 131–160.

Mason BJ, Ritvo EC, Morgan RO, Salvato FR, Goldberg G, Welch B, Mantero-Atienza E. 1994. A double-blind, placebo-controlled pilot study to evaluate the efficacy and safety of oral nalmefene HCl for alcohol dependence. *Alcoholism: Clinical and Experimental Research* 18:1162–1167.

Marlatt GA, Gordon JR. 1985. *Relapse Prevention: Maintenance Strategies in the Treatment of Addictive Behaviors.* New York: Guilford Press.

NIAAA (National Institute on Alcohol Abuse and Alcoholism). 1994a. Twelve step facilitation therapy manual. *Project MATCH Series, Volume 1.* NIH Publication No. 94-3722. Bethesda, MD: NIAAA.

NIAAA. 1994b. Motivational enhancement therapy manual. *Project MATCH Series, Volume 2.* NIH Publication No. 94-3723. Bethesda, MD: NIAAA.

NIAAA. 1995. Cognitive-behavioral coping skills therapy manual. *Project MATCH Series, Volume 3.* NIH Publication No. 95-3911. Bethesda, MD: NIAAA.

Nicoll RA, Alger BE, Jahar C. 1980. Enkephalins block inhibitory pathways in mammalian CNS. *Nature* 287:22–25.

O'Brien CP. 1976. Experimental analysis of conditioning factors in human narcotic addiction. *Pharmacological Reviews* 27:533–543.

O'Brien CP. 1996. Drug addiction and drug abuse. In: Hardman JG, Limbird L, eds. *Goodman and Gilman's The Pharmacologic Basis of Therapeutics.* 9th Edition. New York: McGraw-Hill. Pp. 557–577.

Olds ME, Milner P. 1954. Positive reinforcement produced by electrical stimulation of septal area and other regions of the rat brain. *Journal of Comparative and Physiological Psychology* 47:419–427.

O'Malley SS, Jaffe AJ, Chang G, Rode S, Schottenfeld R, Meyer RE, Rounsaville B. 1996. Six-month follow-up of naltrexone and psychotherapy for alcohol dependence. *Archives of General Psychiatry* 53:217–224.

Phelix CF, Broderick PA. 1995. Light microscopic immunocytochemical evidence of converging serotonin and dopamine terminals in ventrolateral nucleus accumbens. *Brain Research Bulletin* 37:37–40.

Prochaska JO, DiClemente CC. 1986. Toward a comprehensive model of change. In: Miller WR, Heather N, eds. *Treating Addictive Behaviors: Process of Change.* New York: Plenum Press.

Ritz MC, Lamb RJ, Goldberg SR, Kuhar MJ. 1987. Cocaine receptors on dopamine transporters are related to self-administration of cocaine. *Science* 237:1219–1223.

Satel SL, Southwick SM, Gawin FH. 1991. Clinical features of cocaine-induced paranoia. *American Journal of Psychiatry* 148:495–498.

Schuckit MA. 1994. Low level of response to alcohol as a predictor of future alcoholism. *American Journal of Psychiatry* 151:184–189.

Steinberg R, Brun P, Souilhac J, Bougault I, Leyris R, Le Fur G, Soubrie P. 1995. Neurochemical and behavioral effects of neurotensin vs. [D-Tyr[11]]neurotensin on mesolimbic dopaminergic function. *Neuropeptides* 28:42–50.

Tabakoff B, Hoffmann PL. 1996. Alcohol addiction: An enigma among us. *Neuron* 16:909–912.

Thomasson HR, Edenberg HJ, Crabb DW, Mai X-L, Jerome PE, Li T-K, Wang SP, Liu YT, Lu RB, Yin SJ. 1991. Alcohol and aldehyde genotypes and alcoholism in Chinese men. *American Journal of Human Genetics* 48:677–681.

Thomasson HR, Zeng D, Mai X-L, McGarvey S, Deka R, Li T-K. 1994. Population distribution of ADH2 and ALDH2 alleles. *Alcoholism: Clinical and Experimental Research* 18:60A.

Volpicelli JR, Alterman AI, Hayashida M, O'Brien CP. 1992. Naltrexone in the treatment of alcohol dependence. *Archives of General Psychiatry* 46:876–880.

Wafford KA, Whiting PJ. 1992. Ethanol potentiation of $GABA_A$ receptors requires phosphorylation of the alternatively spliced variant of the gamma 2 subunit. *FEBS Letters* 313(2):113–117.

Wafford KA, Burnett DM, Leidenheimer NJ, Burt DR, Want JB, Kofuji P, Dunwiddie TV, Harris RA, Sikela JM. 1991. Ethanol sensitivity of the $GABA_A$ receptor expressed in Xenopus oocytes required 8 amino acids contained in the gamma 2L subunit. *Neuron* 7(1):27–33.

Wilker A. 1973. Dynamics of drug dependence: Implications of a conditioning theory for research and treatment. *Archives of General Psychiatry* 28:611–616.

Wilkinson P, Van Dyke C, Jatlow P, Barash P, Byck R. 1980. Intranasal and oral cocaine kinetics. *Clinical Pharmacology and Therapeutics* 27:386–394.

Wise RA. 1978. Catecholamine theories of reward: A critical review. *Brain Research* 152:215–247.

4

Psychosocial Factors and Prevention

PSYCHOSOCIAL FACTORS

How does use of tobacco, alcohol, opioids, and stimulants begin? Virtually all Americans, some of whom may have a genetic vulnerability to drug abuse, are faced with the decision of whether to smoke, drink alcohol, or take illicit drugs. Why do some individuals say yes and others refuse? Why do some people and not others begin using these drugs in excess and why is it so difficult for some individuals to stop? In addition to studies about genetic vulnerabilities, these and similar questions are the focus of behavioral, epidemiological, and social science research aimed at understanding and preventing drug addiction. The research includes human and animal laboratory studies, and examines such phenomena as environmental factors and personal characteristics that predict addictive behaviors, as well as individual differences in the behavioral mechanisms of drug abuse. This chapter presents a brief overview of key issues in research relevant to the psychosocial and behavioral underpinnings of addiction before presenting examples of the variety of prevention strategies currently used to reduce the prevalence of drug abuse and addiction.

Psychosocial factors include personality and presence of psychiatric disorder, as well as family, peer, and other environmental factors that either increase the risk of an individual developing an addictive disorder (risk factors) or decrease such risks (protective factors). Cognitive and behavioral research is the key to understanding how basic principles of learning and conditioning can be used to modify drug-taking behavior; this research has been reviewed in a variety of reports and monographs (Hawkins et al., 1992; IOM, 1994a,b; IOM, 1996a). Briefly, research indicates that beliefs and attitudes, many of which are learned by watching or listening to role models at home, in the community, or in the media, have a strong influence on drug use and abuse. For example, adolescents typically use drugs when with very close friends, and so the peer influence on drug use and abuse may occur in a cycle: a child chooses friends with similar interests and attitudes, and when one experiments with drugs, the others join in, and soon they are imitating each other's use or abuse. In addition, children are more likely to use drugs if drugs are used by other members of their families. In fact, a family history of drug abuse is the single most important indicator of risk for the children. Although some of this risk may be genetic, it is not clear either to what degree or how genetic vulnerability interacts with environmental factors in such families. The community environment is also crucial; children who live in communities with drugs readily available, drug-using peers, and where drug use is generally accepted are more likely to abuse drugs. Glantz and Pickens (1992) reviewed the literature on vulnerability to drug abuse and found complex relationships among family and community factors. For example, among Mexican Americans, the risks of drug abuse were higher for children from lower socioeconomic group families living in regions with high dropout rates from high school. In contrast, females from families who have a strong identification with Hispanic culture seem to be protected and to engage in drug abuse in lower numbers (Swaim et al., 1993).

Changing the environmental conditions or cues associated with drug use or withdrawal can assist an individual's efforts to abstain from drugs. For example, if drinking a cup of coffee after a meal is associated with smoking, it is important to break that association in the same way that the association between working and smoking is broken when the workplace forbids smoking in one's office. Further, it is well known among treatment providers that patients in recovery from addiction have a higher chance of relapse if they are in environments in which their previous drug use took place, or if they are associating with friends who continue to use drugs.

There has been considerable research on the personalities of alcoholics and individuals addicted to other drugs, but additional multidisciplinary research is needed to identify how specific risk and protective factors interact with biological vulnerability (Hawkins et al., 1992; IOM, 1994a,b; IOM, 1996a). Several studies indicate that children who are less conventional, more tolerant of deviant behavior, less religious, less oriented toward hard work, more rebellious, with lower expectations of academic achievement, and fewer negative beliefs about the harmfulness of drinking and more positive views of the social benefits of drinking are more likely to abuse alcohol as they become older. Similarly, adolescents who are unconventional and have low achievement in school or exhibit problem behaviors are more likely to start to use illicit drugs. Family factors, such as divorce or chronic stress, poor parenting, or a poor child-parent relationship, in addition to parent or sibling use of or attitude toward drugs, also may contribute to drug use.

There is a very high co-occurrence of alcohol and illicit drug dependence with psychiatric disorders, and some experts believe that the drug use amounts to "self-medication" after the psychiatric disorder is manifested (DHHS, 1993). The two most common psychiatric disorders observed in persons with addictive disorders are antisocial personality and depression (Block et al., 1988). In addition, conduct disorder, attention deficit disorder, and anxiety disorders are also associated with an increased risk of drug addition or alcoholism (Kessler et al., 1996). Research suggests that the psychiatric disorder is likely to appear before the drug problem. However, psychiatric problems also can occur after drug use or abuse; thus the precise nature of the co-occurrence of drug problems with other psychiatric illnesses is an important area of research (DHHS, 1993; Kessler et al., 1996).

PREVENTION

In a report focused on prevention of mental disorders, another IOM committee conceptualized new definitions for various levels of prevention interventions and recognized that prevention exists on a continuum with treatment and maintenance (IOM, 1994a). Instead of the classical categories of primary, secondary, and tertiary prevention, the committee defined *universal, selective,* and *indicated* levels of prevention. Universal includes interventions aimed toward an entire population. Selective interventions are those aimed toward individuals who are members of a subgroup or population that is known to be at higher risk for a given disorder, such as aiming interventions at teenagers to prevent drug abuse or drinking. Indicated interventions are for those individuals who exhibit a known risk factor, condition, or abnormality that identifies them as being at high risk for developing a disorder. Indicated interventions, then, could include providing education about alcoholism to young men whose fathers are alcoholics. All three types of interventions are employed to prevent drug abuse and the effectiveness of various approaches is the subject of ongoing research. The rest of this chapter describes some examples of these interventions.

Warning Labels on Alcoholic Beverages

Warning labels on alcoholic beverages, which were required in 1988 by Public Law 100-690, state, "According to the Surgeon General, women should not drink alcoholic beverages during pregnancy because of the risk of birth defects" and "Consumption of alcoholic beverages impairs your ability to drive a car or operate machinery and may cause health problems."

A study of approximately 3,500 pregnant women showed that, after the warning label was introduced, pregnant women who drank very little decreased their alcohol consumption by an average of one ounce of beer per week, whereas pregnant women who drank the equivalent of more than one mixed drink per day did not decrease their alcohol consumption (Hankin, 1994). This study suggests that universal prevention efforts may have some modest success in decreasing the consumption of alcohol, but that more targeted efforts are probably necessary for individuals who are regular users or who are addicted.

An IOM panel on fetal alcohol syndrome found that there are little data on the effectiveness of universal prevention efforts such as warning labels. The panel recommended, however, that these efforts should be continued to raise awareness of the dangers of alcohol, particularly fetal alcohol syndrome and alcohol-related birth defects and neurological defects (IOM, 1996b).

Warning Labels on Tobacco Products

In 1965, Congress passed the first law requiring warning labels on cigarettes (Public Law 89-92). The labels read, "CAUTION: Cigarette Smoking May Be Hazardous to Your Health." This language was strengthened in 1969 to read, "WARNING: The Surgeon General Has Determined that Cigarette Smoking Is Dangerous to Your Health" (Public Law 91-222). In an effort to further strengthen this warning, Congress passed the Comprehensive Smoking Education Act in 1984, which required four different warning labels. One specified the diseases caused by smoking, one urged quitting to improve health; one warned of birth defects and other dangers of smoking while pregnant; and one warned that cigarette smoke contains carbon monoxide (Public Law 98-474).

Labeling changes occurred during a period of increased public information about the dangers of smoking and increasing restrictions on smoking in public places, making it difficult to determine the exact impact of these labeling changes. However, research conducted in Australia before the introduction of cigarette warning labels indicated the importance of varying warning labels so that they would attract attention and ensuring that they are easily understood and easy to see and read (CBRC, 1992).

Advertising Bans

Legal bans or voluntary bans on advertising of alcohol and tobacco also represent a prevention effort; they curb exposure to messages that encourage alcohol and nicotine use. Cigarette advertising has been banned from radio and television since 1969, and advertisements for little cigars were similarly banned in 1973 (Public Laws 91-222 and 93-109). As of 1996, 48 states had some type of restriction, from minimal to comprehensive, on smoking in public places (CHS, 1996). In 1996, the liquor industry ended a self-imposed ban on television advertising. This action spurred debate about whether there should be comprehensive regulation of alcohol advertising along the lines of that imposed on the tobacco industry.

Cigarette Promotions

Despite the ban on radio and television advertising, the tobacco industry spends approximately $4.5 billion each year on billboard and other advertising aimed at promoting consumption, approximately quadrupling their expenditures since 1980 (IOM, 1994b). Cigarette advertising uses images to portray smokers as independent, healthy, adventure-seeking, and attractive (IOM, 1994b). However, the vast majority of marketing dollars are spent on promotional activities, such as sponsoring sports events and public entertainment and distributing T-shirts, hats, and other items that provide free advertising by prominently displaying the companies'' logos. A study of 166 televised sports events indicates that the TV audience is exposed to tobacco advertising through stadium signs and brief verbal or visual product sponsorships (Madden and Grube, 1994). There is increasing concern that advertisements and promotional activities are aimed at encouraging children to smoke, and there is research evidence to support that perception. For example, Camel Cigarettes' advertisements featuring a cartoon character, Joe Camel, greatly increased Camel's market share among children, and studies suggest that participation in promotional activities (e.g., owning a promotional item) is strongly associated with a higher risk of tobacco use among adolescents (IOM, 1994b; Altman et al., 1996).

Research on the effects of legal restrictions on promotional activities has been conducted in many countries. A study of 33 countries concluded that total advertising bans resulted in decreases in consumption that occurred four times faster than decreases following partial bans, whereas consumption increased in countries with no advertising restrictions (IOM, 1994b).

In August 1996, the FDA issued final regulations aimed at decreasing advertising to young people. The new rule will ban brand-name sponsorship of sporting or other events, cars, or teams, and ban brand names on hats, T-shirts, gym bags, and other products. The rule also limits advertising in publications with at least 2 million youthful readers or where at least 15 percent of the readership is youths, permits black-and-white text only, bans billboards within 1,000 feet of schools and playgrounds, and restricts most other outdoor advertising to black-and-white text only.

Alcohol Promotions

Approximately $1 billion is spent every year to advertise alcoholic beverages, generally portraying drinking as a healthy, attractive, and success-oriented activity (IOM, 1989). A study of 166 televised sports events indicated that commercials advertising alcoholic beverages were aired more than any other product (Madden and Grube, 1994). During the 1996 Olympic Games, Budweiser beer TV commercials featured bullfrog characters, which Mothers Against Drunk Driving (MADD) criticized as aimed at a very young audience (Batog, 1996). An August 1996 marketing survey indicated that most children between 6 and 11 years of age recognized the bullfrogs. The impact of these and other advertisements on consumption is not clear, but there is evidence that advertisements tend to stimulate consumption of the products in general, not just the specific product advertised (IOM, 1989).

Advertisements and commercials are not the only way that the media influence drug use. "Social learning theory" predicts that viewers will "model" attractive TV or film characters who smoke or drink, resulting in viewers having more positive attitudes toward these drugs and increasing their consumption (IOM, 1989). Recent analyses of prime-time television programs found that two-thirds of the programs made references to alcohol and half portrayed consumption of alcohol, averaging more than eight drinking acts per hour (Wallach et al., 1990). In that study, alcohol was consumed by affluent professionals and portrayed in a positive way; alcohol problems were clearly depicted in only 10 percent of the episodes. Television programs could therefore encourage drinking among viewers; this seems especially likely among adolescents, because they watch a lot of television and movies and tend to imitate the clothes, expressions, and behaviors they see in the media. The portrayal of smoking on TV, and in music videos and films could have a similar effect. Although there is no conclusive research in this area, social scientists presume that the consumption behaviors portrayed in such media programming have an impact similar to advertising, which has been extensively studied.

Restrictions on Smoking in Specific Locations

Smoking was first banned on U.S. domestic airline flights of two hours or less in 1987. This was later extended to flights of six hours or less in 1989, and in 1995 a treaty between Canada, the United States, and Australia banned smoking on all nonstop flights between the countries (Public Laws 100-202 and 101-164 and ICAO, 1995). Many international airlines also voluntarily ban smoking on some or all flights.

Smoking was first banned from clinic areas that administered some federal programs in 1993 (Public Law 103-11); this was extended to schools, day care centers, and libraries receiving federal funds in 1994 (Public Law 103-227), and many federal agencies now ban smoking in their buildings. The private sector also restricts or bans smoking in many other buildings, including hospitals, office buildings, and restaurants. Smoking bans in the workplace have been associated with significant decreases in smoking during work hours (Stave and Jackson, 1991; Daughton et al., 1992) and significant decreases in nonsmokers' exposure to environmental tobacco smoke (Borland et al., 1991; Hammond et al., 1995). There is mixed evidence as to whether bans result in higher quit rates; two studies have found positive effects of such bans (Longo et al., 1996; Stave and Jackson, 1991), but others have found no effect (Daughton et al., 1992).

Prices and Use

The federal government taxes tobacco products and alcoholic beverages, and all the states have additional taxes on these products (IOM, 1989; DHHS, 1991). Raising the costs of legal drugs such as alcohol and cigarettes has been shown to decrease use. For example, the consumption of alcoholic beverages is reduced when prices are increased (IOM, 1989). This is especially likely for youth (one study found that a 10-cent increase in the price of beer resulted in a 15 percent decrease in the numbers of youths who drink 3 to 5 beers each day, while a 30-cent increase in the price of distilled spirits resulted in a 27 percent decline in the numbers of youths who were heavy drinkers of liquor [Grossman et al., 1987]). As a result, taxes have the potential for decreasing consumption. Although taxes have tended to increase over the years, they have not risen nearly as much as other increases in cost; for example, in 1990 federal taxes accounted for 11 percent of the cost of cigarettes to consumers, compared to 37 percent in 1950.

In contrast to efforts to decrease consumption, "happy hour" promotions at bars and restaurants, which offer discounts on drinks or free food with drinks, resulted in increased consumption in barroom and restaurant settings (Babor et al., 1980).

In 1988, California voters passed Proposition 99, which increased the tax on a package of cigarettes from 10 cents to 35 cents (Tobacco Education Oversight Committee, 1993). Twenty percent of the funds from the tax were allocated to anti-tobacco education in schools and communities. Studies have shown a clear effect on consumption of the resulting increased per pack price of cigarettes. For example, the month the increase went into effect, there was a 25 percent decline in cigarette consumption (Hu et al., 1994) and it is estimated that sales were reduced by 819 million packs between 1990 and 1992 (Hu et al., 1995). Between 1988 and 1992, the proportion of Californians ages 20 and older who smoked dropped from 27 percent to 20 percent and cigarette consumption (defined as the number of packs sold per civilian adult) decreased by 14 percent (Tobacco Education Oversight Committee, 1993). Unfortunately, there were no differences in smoking behavior for adolescents ages 12 to 17. In contrast, prior to 1988 nationwide smoking during those years increased followed by smaller decreases from 1988 to 1992 for adults, and statistically significant decreases for adolescents.

In Canada, similar decreases in the prevalence of smoking followed a substantial increase in cigarette taxes, one even greater than that in California. The prevalence of smoking among adults dropped from 36 percent to 26 percent between 1981 and 1991 when the taxes were significantly raised, and the proportion of adolescents ages 15 to 19 who smoked daily plummeted from 40 percent to 16 percent (Sweanor et al., 1993). Although there is no way to determine the extent to which decreases in adult smoking in California or Canada can be attributed to the higher costs of cigarettes or the public education program, the results suggest that when taxes are raised, and the resulting revenues used for public education campaigns, there can be considerable benefit to public health (Sweanor et al., 1992; Thompson, 1994). A study in Great Britain showed that both women and men in lower socioeconomic groups were more sensitive to the price of cigarettes than to health publicity campaigns, and that women were more sensitive to price in general than were men (Townsend et al., 1994).

Access/Server Intervention

Access to alcohol and cigarettes can be limited in a variety of ways. Decisions about the locations of liquor stores, the granting of liquor licenses to restaurants, the training of bartenders and waiters to limit alcohol consumption, and the locations of cigarette vending machines and cigarettes in stores can all serve to limit access.

There is statistical evidence of an association between the number of outlets that sell alcoholic beverages and the levels of alcohol consumption and alcohol-related deaths (DHHS, 1993). However, more research is needed to determine if the increased availability of alcohol is responsible.

Server intervention seeks to reduce a customer's likelihood of intoxication or driving while intoxicated by influencing the incentives and behaviors of those serving beverages. For example, servers can be trained to promote nonalcoholic beverages and food or to delay serving an alcoholic beverage if it would be likely to intoxicate the patron. There is some research evidence that these interventions are effective (IOM, 1989). In addition, a bar or restaurant can charge more for alcoholic drinks than soft drinks, serve smaller drinks, and stop selling pitchers of beer.

The newly completed FDA regulations will, among other measures, ban cigarette vending machines and self-service displays except in nightclubs and other facilities that are totally inaccessible to persons under 18. Such a ban has been characterized as a law enforcement approach to reduce access to tobacco by children and youth and studies suggest that a law enforcement approach by itself may not be effective (DiFranza et al., 1996; Feighery et al., 1991). In addition, some have argued that the focus on youth access and law enforcement may have unintended consequences in part by emphasizing that smoking is for adults—therefore, something for adolescents to aspire to (Glantz, 1996). Most agree, however, that approaches to reduce access are necessary to a comprehensive strategy to reduce nicotine addiction in young people (IOM, 1994b). Thus, the impact of these new regulations will be a fruitful area of future research to determine which of their components are the most effective.

The Role of Primary Care Physicians

Primary care physicians represent another set of actors in the strategy for nearly universal prevention efforts. It is known that brief interventions by physicians can be quite effective in stimulating people to quit smoking or reduce their alcohol consumption (Ockene et al., 1991, 1994; Bien et al., 1993; Kahan et al., 1995; Fiore et al., 1990; Sachs, 1990). Most children and adults are seen by a primary care physician at least occasionally, and physicians have been encouraged by the federal government to ask patients about their smoking, drinking, and use of illicit drugs. These questions give physicians the opportunity to share information about the health risks of these behaviors.

Integrating diagnosis, treatment, and prevention of addictive disorders into primary care settings is challenging, however, and often this integrative strategy is not provided by increasingly overburdened primary care physicians. In 1994, a major conference was held to explore this issue and participants found that this resistance was a result of a lack of appropriate training, negative attitudes of physicians about addictive disorders, and lack of time (Josiah Macy, Jr. Foundation, 1994). The participants, citing the cost of undiagnosed and untreated addictive disorders as almost $240 billion a year, made a series of recommendations to increase training and competencies of primary care physicians through changes in certifying medical board and accreditation councils, among other mechanisms. Achieving such a change in practice patterns will require not only training, but also further demonstrations of the effectiveness of these approaches. Although evidence exists that physician intervention increases the chances of abstinence from alcohol or tobacco, more research is needed on the ways in which physician interventions can be an effective prevention strategy.

School-Based Prevention Programs

Schools are the site of most programs designed to prevent drug abuse and addiction, and these programs have been systematically evaluated for almost two decades (IOM, 1996a). In recent years, large numbers of these studies have been evaluated together in meta-analyses aimed at determining patterns of effectiveness of various types of programs. For example, Tobler conducted a meta-analysis of 143 school-based drug programs (including nicotine) for students in grades 6 through 12, which he categorized into five types: informational programs about drug effects; programs that focused on enhancing self-esteem or general competence rather than knowledge about drugs; knowledge plus self-esteem; programs that focused on peer interaction; and programs that took place outside the school. The meta-analysis indicated that peer programs were the most likely to decrease later drug use, and that knowledge plus self-esteem programs and the programs outside the school also had some impact (Tobler, 1986, 1989). Tobler later re-analyzed the data, eliminating the weakest programs, and found that neither knowledge-only, self-esteem-only, nor knowledge plus self-esteem programs prevented drug use, whereas peer programs still were most effective and programs outside the school were moderately effective. Upon closer examination, Tobler concluded that the use of mental health professionals or counselors accounted for the peer programs' effectiveness.

Bangert-Drowns conducted a meta-analysis on 33 programs, limiting his analysis to programs in schools with "traditional students," and eliminating any tobacco-only programs (NRC, 1993). Most of the programs were knowledge-only or knowledge plus self-esteem programs, usually led by teachers. The programs significantly increased knowledge and changed attitudes, but they did not affect behavior. He also found that the lecture format was the weakest and peer leaders were more effective than adults.

The most widely disseminated school-based drug abuse prevention program in the nation is D.A.R.E. (Drug Abuse Resistance Education), but evaluations of these programs consistently show they have no long-term effects (Ennett et al., 1994a,b).

Effective Programs

Two school-based prevention programs have demonstrated long-term success: Life Skills Training and the Midwestern Project (IOM, 1996a). **Life Skills Training** is designed for seventh graders, with "booster sessions" in eighth and ninth grades. The program has been rigorously evaluated in 150 junior high schools in New York and New Jersey that serve primarily white middle-class students. Four-year follow-up results show that rates of smoking and marijuana use were one-half to three-quarters lower among students who participated, with more modest decreases in use of alcohol (Falco, 1992). Six-year follow-up showed significant decreases in use and heavy use of cigarettes and alcohol, but not in use of illegal drugs (IOM, 1996a). **The Midwestern Project** is a 10-session, school-based social skills and peer-resistance skills curriculum, supplemented by parental involvement, media campaigns, and training of community leaders (IOM, 1996a). An evaluation after six years found that the program significantly decreased the use of cigarettes, alcohol, marijuana, and cocaine for high-risk and low-risk students (Pentz et al., 1989a,b).

Family-Based Interventions

Although poor parenting causes many of the problems associated with children's drug abuse, there are few studies and as yet no evidence that family-based interventions alone are successful in preventing drug abuse (IOM, 1996a). However, one study found lower rates of alcohol initiation when parent training was used in conjunction with modified teaching practices (IOM, 1996a).

Media-Based Prevention Interventions

The positive portrayal of smoking and alcohol use on TV programs and in movies has been seen as a major influence on attitudes toward the use of these drugs. Efforts to use television overtly to counteract those messages have been made repeatedly over the years.

Public service announcements and other media-based interventions are relatively inexpensive efforts to attempt to influence the knowledge and attitudes of a large number of children and youth. However, there are no rigorous studies of their impact on the audience's later drug use or abuse. Media interventions aimed at preventing adolescent smoking have been found to affect knowledge and, in some cases, attitudes, but have not shown a sustained impact on behavior (IOM, 1996a; Murray et al., 1994). However, TV anti-smoking messages have been found to be effective in combination with school-based programs at preventing or limiting adolescent smoking behavior (Flynn et al., 1992).

Laws to Prevent Teen Alcohol Use and Smoking

Epidemiological and public health research has been conducted in states and communities that have enacted new laws or policies to prevent or limit adolescent drinking and smoking by raising the age at which an individual can buy alcohol and tobacco products. The research examines how the environment, including the cost and availability of drugs, influences the likelihood of addiction and related problems.

In 1983, Hingson et al. published a seminal study that evaluated the impact of raising the legal drinking age in Massachusetts from 18 to 20. They compared drinking, drinking and driving, and nonfatal accidents in Massachusetts and New York, which kept its drinking age at 18. Results indicated that the law was unevenly enforced, but that nighttime single-vehicle fatal car crashes declined more for 18- and 19-year-olds in Massachusetts than they did in New York (Waller, 1995). Other studies in different states clearly indicated that raising the legal drinking age decreased teenage drinking and driving and involvement in drinking-related car crashes (Waller, 1995). Despite these positive effects, it is not clear that laws restricting sales of alcohol to minors have actually reduced access. One large survey study, for example, has shown that, in 1995, 75 percent of eighth graders and 90 percent of tenth graders reported that it was easy to obtain alcohol (Johnston et al., 1996).

Research on the effect of laws restricting tobacco sales to minors has been reviewed by another IOM committee (IOM, 1994a). By 1990, 45 states and the District of Columbia had legislation that prevented minors' access to tobacco products, but these laws were rarely enforced (DHHS, 1991). For example, in one Massachusetts community, an 11-year-old girl purchased cigarettes in 75 of her 100 attempts to do so (DiFranza et al., 1987). Several studies of young teenagers had similar results (DHHS, 1991). As discussed above, the new FDA regulations include legal sanctions for sale of tobacco to minors, along with other mechanisms to reduce youth access to tobacco, such as banning vending machine sales under certain circumstances (Kessler et al., 1996; Kessler et al., 1997). Because these approaches are similar to those taken for alcohol, some have argued that their effectiveness may be less than anticipated and, thus, the opportunity now exists for renewed evaluation of their efficacy.

CONCLUSION

Some of the key research challenges to be addressed in the area of psychosocial factors of addiction and prevention are listed in Table 4.1. Although we are now aware of many environmental risk factors for the development of drug abuse and addiction, a greater understanding of the relative strength of specific risk factors and what factors may protect individuals from addiction, is needed (Appendix H). Interdisciplinary research is also necessary to understand the relationships and interactions among specific risk and protective factors. Increased knowledge in these areas will not only help protect the health of individuals, but could also be used to design more effective preventive interventions to improve public health. Further research on existing preventive interventions is also needed. Although a rich and varied set of interventions is available, their effectiveness is sometimes unknown, particularly in special populations such as rural youth, minority groups, and others. Meeting these challenges and integrating research findings from these and other disciplines should be an area of high national priority to strengthen a science-based approach to the reduction of drug abuse and addiction.

TABLE 4.1 Some Future Challenges in Psychosocial and Prevention Research

- Examination of both the risk and protective environmental factors that are important in determining an individual's vulnerability to drug abuse or addiction
- Examination of environmental and behavioral factors that are important in the development of addiction following initial or social use of drugs and alcohol
- Examination of the relationship of drug abuse with other psychiatric disorders
- Examination of relationship among alcohol abuse and the abuse of cocaine, nicotine, opioids, and other drugs
- Investigation of strategies to identify at-risk youth and involve them in effective prevention programs
- Development of effective prevention strategies for pregnant women who may drink alcohol or abuse drugs
- Continued evaluation of prevention strategies aimed at reducing HIV transmission from needle sharing and other behaviors associated with drug abuse
- Development and evaluation of methods to prevent smoking initiation and nicotine dependence in children and youth
- Examination of the personality/temperament, as well as physiological and biochemical, attributes of resilient children from families with a history of drug abuse or alcoholism
- Investigation of factors that affect the success of advertising bans and increased taxes in the prevention of alcoholism and nicotine addiction
- Evaluation of effects of regulation of nicotine on prevalence of nicotine addiction and smoking cessation rates among populations differing in age, gender, ethnicity, economic status, or other variables
- Evaluation of methods designed for use by primary care providers to assess risks of alcoholism and drug abuse in their patients
- Examination of school-based prevention activities and the variables that may limit or augment their effectiveness
- Review of the adequacy of existing national data sets to determine prevalence of drug abuse and alcoholism, particularly among youth

REFERENCES

Altman DG, Levine DW, Coeytaux R, Slade J, Jaffe R. 1996. Tobacco promotion and susceptibility to tobacco use among adolescents aged 12 through 17 years in a nationally representative sample. *American Journal of Public Health* 86:1590–1593.

Babor TF, Mendelson JH, Uhly B, Souza E. 1980. Drinking patterns in experimental and barroom settings. *Journal of Studies on Alcohol* 41(7):635–651.

Batog J. 1996. MADD demands Bud drop frog ads. *Washington Post*. September 13.

Bien TH, Miller WR, Tonigan JS. 1993. Brief interventions for alcohol problems. A review. *Addiction* 88:315–336.

Block J, Block J, Keyes S. 1988. Longitudinally foretelling drug usage in adolescence: Early childhood personality and environmental precursors. *Child Development* 59:336–355.

Borland R, Owen N, Hill D, Schofield P. 1991. Predicting attempts and sustained cessation of smoking after the introduction of workplace smoking bans. *Health Psychology* 10(5):336–342.

CBRC (Centre for Behavioural Research in Cancer). 1992. *Health Warnings and Contents Labeling on Tobacco Products.* Australia: Centre for Behavioural Research in Cancer.

CHS (Coalition on Smoking or Health). 1996. *State Legislated Actions on Tobacco Issues at-a-Glance.* Washington, DC: Coalition on Smoking or Health. March.

Daughton DM, Andrews CE, Orona CP, Patil KD, Rennard SI. 1992. Total indoor smoking ban and smoker behavior. *Preventive Medicine* 21(5):670–676.

DHHS (U.S. Department of Health and Human Services). 1991. *Strategies to Control Tobacco Use in the United States: A Blueprint for Public Health Action in the 1990s.* Smoking and Tobacco Control Monographs 1. Rockville, MD: National Cancer Institute, U.S. Department of Health and Human Services. October.

DHHS. 1993. *Eighth Special Report to the U.S. Congress on Alcohol and Health.* NIH Publication No. 94-3699. Rockville, MD: National Institute on Alcohol Abuse and Alcoholism, U.S. Department of Health and Human Services. September.

DiFranza JR, Norwood BD, Garner DW, Tye JB. 1987. Legislative efforts to protect children from tobacco. *Journal of the American Medical Association* 263:2784–2787.

DiFranza JR, Savageau JA, Aisquith BF. 1996. Youth access to tobacco: The effects of age, gender, vending machine locks, and "It's the Law" programs. *American Journal of Public Health* 86:221–224.

Ennett ST, Rosenbaum DP, Flewelling RL, Bieler GS, Ringwalt CR, Bailey SL. 1994a. Long-term evaluation of Drug Abuse Resistance Education. *Addictive Behaviors* 19:113–125.

Ennett ST, Tobler NS, Ringwalt CL, Flewelling RL. 1994b. How effective is Drug Abuse Resistance Education? A meta-analysis of project DARE outcome evaluations. *American Journal of Public Health* 84(9):1394–1401.

Falco M. 1992. *The Making of a Drug-Free America: Programs That Work.* New York: Times Books.

Feighery E, Altman DG, Shaffer G. 1991. The effects of combining education and enforcement to reduce tobacco sales to minors. A study of four northern California communities. *Journal of the American Medical Association* 266(22):3186–3188.

Fiore MC, Pierce JP, Remington PL, Fiore BJ. 1990. Cigarette cessation: The clinician's role in cessation, prevention, and public health. *Disease-a-Month* 36(4):181–242.

Flynn BS, Worden JK, Secker-Walker RH, Badger GJ, Geller BM, Costanza MC. 1992. Prevention of cigarette smoking through mass media intervention and school programs. *American Journal of Public Health* 82(6):827–834.

Glantz SA. 1996. Preventing Tobacco Use—The Youth Access Trap. [Editorial]. *American Journal of Public Health* 86(2): 156–158.

Glantz M, Pickens R. 1992. *Vulnerability to Drug Abuse.* Washington, DC: American Psychological Press.

Grossman M, Coate D, Arluck GM. 1987. Price sensitivity of alcoholic beverages in the United States: Youth alcohol consumption. In: Holder HD, ed. *Control Issues in Alcohol Abuse Prevention: Strategies for States and Communities.* Greenwich, CT: JAI Press. Pp. 169–198.

Hammond SK, Sorensen G, Youngstrom R, Ockene JK. 1995. Occupational exposure to environmental tobacco smoke. *Journal of the American Medical Association* 274(12):956–960.

Hankin JR. 1994. FAS prevention strategies: Passive and active measures. *Alcohol Health and Research World* 18:62–66.

Hawkins JD, Catalano RF, Miller JY. 1992. Risk and protective factors for alcohol and other drug problems in adolescence and early adulthood: Implications for substance abuse prevention. *Psychological Bulletin* 112(1):64–105.

Hingson RW, Scotch N, Mangione T, Meyers A, Glantz L, Heeren T, Lin N, Mucatel M, Pierce G. 1983. Impact of legislation raising the legal drinking age in Massachusetts from 18 to 20. *American Journal of Public Health* 73(2):163–170.

Hu TW, Bai J, Keeler ET, Barnett PG, Sung HY. 1994. The impact of California Proposition 99, a major anti-smoking law, on cigarette consumption. *Journal of Public Health Policy* 15(1):26–36.

Hu TW, Sung HY, Keeler TE. 1995. Reducing cigarette consumption in California: Tobacco taxes vs. an anti-smoking media campaign. *American Journal of Public Health* 85(9):1218–1222.

ICAO (International Civil Aviation Organization). 1995. *Agreement to Ban Smoking on International Passenger Flights*. Montreal, Canada: International Civil Aviation Organization.

IOM (Institute of Medicine). 1989. *Prevention and Treatment of Alcohol Problems: Research Opportunities*. Washington, DC: National Academy Press.

IOM. 1994a. *Reducing Risks for Mental Disorders: Frontiers for Preventive Intervention Research*. Washington, DC: National Academy Press.

IOM. 1994b. *Growing Up Tobacco Free*. Washington, DC: National Academy Press.

IOM. 1996a. *Pathways of Addiction: Opportunities in Drug Abuse Research*. Washington, DC: National Academy Press.

IOM. 1996b. *Fetal Alcohol Syndrome: Diagnosis, Epidemiology, Prevention, and Treatment*. Washington, DC: National Academy Press.

Johnston LD, O'Malley PM, Bachman JG. 1996. *National Survey Results on Drug Use from the Monitoring the Future Survey, 1975–1996*. Ann Arbor, MI: Institute for Social Research, University of Michigan.

Josiah Macy, Jr. Foundation. 1994. *Training about Alcohol and Substance Abuse for All Primary Care Physicians. Proceedings of a Conference, October 2–5*. New York: Josiah Macy, Jr. Foundation.

Kahan M, Wilson L, Becker L. 1995. Effectiveness of physician-based interventions with problem drinkers: A review. *Canadian Medical Association Journal* 152(6):851–859.

Kessler DA, Witt AM, Barnett PS, Zeller MR, Natanblut SL, Wilkenfeld JP, Lorraine CC, Thompson LJ, Schultz WB. 1996. The Food and Drug Administration's regulation of tobacco products. *The New England Journal of Medicine* 335(13):988–994.

Kessler DA, Barnett PS, Witt A, Zeller MR, Mande JR, Schultz WB. 1997. The legal and scientific basis for FDA's assertion of jurisdiction over cigarettes and smokeless tobacco products. *Journal of the American Medical Association* 277(5):405–409.

Longo DR, Brownson RC, Johnson JC, Hewett JE, Kruse RL, Novotny TE, Logan RA. 1996. Hospital smoking bans and employee smoking behavior: Results of a national survey. *Journal of the American Medical Association* 275(16):1252–1257.

Madden PA, Grube JW. 1994. The frequency and nature of alcohol and tobacco advertis-
ing in televised sports, 1990 through 1992. *American Journal of Public Health*
84(2):297–299.
Murray DM, Prokhorov AV, Harty KC. 1994. Effects of a statewide anti-smoking cam-
paign on mass media messages and smoking beliefs. *Preventive Medicine* 23(1):54–
60.
NRC (National Research Council). 1993. *Preventing Drug Abuse: What Do We Know?*
Washington, DC: National Academy Press.
Ockene JK, Kristeller J, Goldberg R, Amick TL, Pekow PS, Hosmer D, Quirk M, Kalan
K. 1991. Increasing the efficiency of physician-delivered smoking interventions: A
randomized clinical trial. *Journal of General Internal Medicine* 6(1):1–8.
Ockene JK, Kristeller J, Pbert L, Herbert JR, Luippold R, Goldberg RJ, Landon J, Kalan
K. 1994. The physician-delivered smoking intervention project: Can short-term in-
terventions produce long-term effects for a general outpatient population? *Health
Psychology* 13(3):278–281.
Pentz MA, Dwyer J, MacKinnon D, Flay BR, Hansen WB, Wang EY, Johnson CA.
1989a. A multi-community trial for primary prevention of adolescent drug abuse.
Journal of the American Medical Association 261:3259–3266.
Pentz MA, MacKinnon D, Flay B, Hansen W, Johnson CA, Dwyer J. 1989b. Primary
prevention of chronic diseases in adolescence: Effects of the midwestern prevention
project on tobacco use. *American Journal of Epidemiology* 130:713–724.
Sachs DP. 1990. Smoking cessation strategies: What works, what doesn't. *Journal of the
American Dental Association* Suppl:13S–19S.
Stave GM, Jackson GW. 1991. Effect of a total work-site smoking ban on employee
smoking and attitudes. *Journal of Occupational Medicine* 33(8):884–890.
Swaim RC, Oetting ER, Thurman PJ, Beauvais F, Edwards R. 1993. American Indian
adolescent drug use and socialization characteristics: A cross-cultural comparison.
Journal of Cross Cultural Psychology 24(1):53–70.
Sweanor D, Ballin S, Corcoran R, Davis A, Deasy K, Ferrence R, Lahey R, Lucido S,
Nethery WJ, Wasserman J. 1993. Report of the Tobacco Research Study Group on
tobacco pricing and taxation in the United States. *Tobacco Control* (Suppl) 1:S31–
S36.
Sweanor D, Martial L, Dossetor J. 1992. *The Canadian Tobacco Tax Increase: A Case
Study.* Ottawa, Ontario: The Non-Smokers' Rights Association and The Smoking
and Health Action Foundation.
Thompson B. 1994. Research in tobacco use prevention: Where should we go next? *Pre-
ventive Medicine* 23:676–682.
Tobacco Education Oversight Committee. 1993. *Toward a Tobacco-Free California:
Exploring a New Frontier, 1993–1995.* Sacramento, CA: Tobacco Education Over-
sight Committee, February.
Tobler NS. 1986. Meta-analysis of 143 adolescent drug prevention programs: Quantita-
tive outcome results of program participants compared to a control or comparison
group. *Journal of Drug Issues* 16(4):537–567.
Tobler NS. 1989. *Drug Prevention Programs Can Work: Research Findings.* Albany:
School of Social Welfare, State University of New York, Albany. Unpublished.
Townsend J, Roderick P, Cooper J. 1994. Cigarette smoking by socioeconomic group,
sex, and age: Effects of price, income, and health publicity. *British Medical Journal*
309:923–927.

Wagenaar AC, Finnegan JR, Wolfson M, Anstine PS, Williams CL, Perry CL. 1993. Where and how adolescents obtain alcoholic beverages. *Public Health Report* 108(4):459–464.

Wallach L, Grube JW, Madden PA, Breed W. 1990. Portrayals of alcohol on prime-time television. *Journal of Studies on Alcohol* 51(5):428–437.

Waller PF. 1995. Commentary: Legislation raising the legal drinking age in Massachusetts. *Alcohol Health and Research World* 19(1):52–53.

5

Treating Addictive Disorders

One of the most enduring myths about addiction is that treatment for these disorders is ineffective. This chapter provides a brief overview of the variety of types of treatments available, what is known about their effectiveness, and some questions that require further research. As previous chapters have described, addiction involves a complex interplay of biological, social, and individual factors. This interplay complicates treatment in much the same way that treatment for diabetes or hypertension is complicated by disease severity, the individual's motivation and ability to control diet or exercise levels, social support, and other factors.

O'Brien and McLellan (1996) reviewed and compared treatment literature for addictive disorders and three common health problems—hypertension, diabetes, and asthma. Treatment effectiveness for addiction was defined as a 50 percent reduction in drug taking after six months. The literature reviewed showed treatment for alcoholism to be successful for 40 percent to 70 percent of patients; success rates for cocaine addiction were 50 percent to 60 percent, opioids 50 percent to 80 percent, and nicotine 20 percent to 40 percent. Interestingly, review of studies relevant to diabetes, hypertension, and asthma revealed that high proportions of these patients did not follow their physicians' advice and did not adhere to diet and other behavioral components of their treatment. For example, among patients with insulin-dependent diabetes, less than 50 percent adhered to their medication regimen and less than 30 percent conformed to their diet and other self-care requirements. Less than 30 percent of patients with asthma or hypertension were found to take their medications as instructed. Noncompliance and other factors, according to the studies reviewed, resulted in 50 percent to 60 percent of hypertension and 60 to 80 percent of asthma patients needing to be retreated within a year.

The comparability of these data argue that addiction is similar to these three common medical illnesses in that they all can be treated successfully in many patients, but none can be cured and all four often require retreatment. Yet, there are important differences between addiction and these other illnesses in the perception of the public, insurance companies, and physicians. Few would argue that retreatment for diabetes, hypertension, or asthma indicates treatment failure, or that retreatment should be withheld from or denied to these patients when they relapse and their symptoms reoccur. Yet such an argument is commonly made about addiction.

Similar to the treatment of many illnesses, addiction treatment involves three major stages—detoxification (or acute stabilization), rehabilitation, and follow-up care (McLellan et al., 1997). For all addictive disorders, the initial treatment goal is to help the person stop using alcohol, nicotine, cocaine, heroin, or other drugs and to begin to address the person's physiological, emotional, and motivational status. Detoxification can be accomplished in a variety of ways, depending on the drug(s) involved. For example, treatment of alcoholism usually requires complete abstinence from drinking, but treatment of heroin addiction often utilizes methadone as a substitute to achieve a gradual withdrawal and detoxification.

The rehabilitation phase of treatment continues the treatment components utilized initially, but can include additional components, such as education about the harmful effects of drugs and ways to avoid relapse, as well as behavioral or other types of therapy. Participation in support groups is also a common element of the rehabilitation phase. Follow-up or aftercare is the final phase of treatment for addiction. Aftercare varies considerably in terms of length and frequency of interventions, but prevention of relapse is the major goal of all aftercare strategies.

Relapse is the single most important target of addiction treatment. Data from clinical and outcomes research have shown that many types of treatment approaches are effective in reducing drug use and improving health, but that long-term abstinence is difficult to achieve (McLellan et al., 1995). McLellan and colleagues also found that the longer a person is in treatment, the more likely the treatment will be successful. A critical period seems to be the early stages of treatment, during which attrition is high. Additionally, the literature review provided a strong indication that treatment programs offering a greater variety of services (e.g., counseling, job training, housing assistance, and other services) targeted to an individual's specific problems tend to be most effective.

Despite the general effectiveness of addiction treatment, there is tremendous variation in the types of services offered, and considerable variation in the amount of information available regarding the effectiveness of the major types of treatment programs or any specific individual programs. In part, the variety reflects different approaches that have developed over time to address addiction to specific drugs (e.g., heroin vs. alcohol). In addition, not all strategies can be employed for specific addictions. For example, there are successful replacement pharmacotherapies available for heroin and nicotine addiction (methadone and nicotine gum or patches), but not for alcohol or cocaine. Often, however, treatment approaches are based on underlying assumptions and viewpoints regarding the causes of addiction, ranging from addiction as a disease to addiction as a moral failure.

The remainder of this chapter describes some of the various approaches taken, the relevant knowledge base, and the gaps in knowledge about treatment of alcohol and cocaine addiction first, followed by treatment for opioid addiction, and concludes with a description of some new advances in treatment for nicotine addiction. Some of the information in these sections overlaps, because there are certain elements common to all addiction treatment. However, it is important to keep in mind that success and failure in treatment involve both treatment factors (e.g., setting, length, intensity) and patient factors (e.g., severity of addiction, presence of other psychiatric and medical conditions, social support, education, and readiness for change). Although much is known about the general effectiveness of addiction treatment, the interaction of specific treatment factors with specific patient factors, often called patient-treatment matching, is an area of great interest in research.

TREATMENTS FOR ALCOHOL AND COCAINE ADDICTION

Treatment Setting

One of the variables in addiction treatment that is the subject of considerable research is the setting in which the treatment occurs. In general, these settings include inpatient versus outpatient settings, but outpatient settings also vary in their intensity and range from regular visits to a clinic to prolonged participation in day hospital programs. Treatment for alcoholism has been shaped in part by the legality of alcohol use, the predominance of Alcoholics Anonymous groups, and the availability of private insurance for many patients, leading to programs based on an initial hospital stay; whereas treatments for addiction to illegal drugs, such as heroin and cocaine, has developed largely with public funding, leading to a greater reliance on outpatient care and therapeutic communities. However, particularly for cocaine, these distinctions are blurring, which reflects the reality that many people addicted to one drug often are addicted to or abuse other drugs as well. This section emphasizes treatment approaches used for alcohol and cocaine addiction, because treatment of opioid addiction involves some significant differences discussed later in the chapter.

TABLE 5.1 Duration of Addiction Treatment

Treatment Setting	Duration
Detoxification/stabilization (if necessary)	3–5 days
Inpatient, hospital-based programs	7–11 days
Residential, non-hospital programs	30–90 days
Therapeutic community programs	6 months–2 years
Outpatient, abstinence-oriented programs	30–120 days
Intensive outpatient	Begin at full or half days 5 times per week for one month, gradually decreasing
Aftercare (biweekly or monthly group meetings)	2 years
Maintenance treatments (e.g., methadone)	Years–lifetime

SOURCE: McLellan et al. (1997).

Decisions about treatment setting ideally take into account the overall status of the patient, and much work has been done to help guide such decisions. For example, the American Society of Addiction Medicine recently published a second edition of its *Patient Placement Criteria* (1997) which presents separate guidelines for adults and adolescents and defines five levels of service for each: early intervention, outpatient services, intensive outpatient/partial hospitalization services, residential/inpatient services, and medically managed intensive inpatient services. Table 5.1 summarizes the average length of treatment in various settings.

The American Psychiatric Association (1995) has published a set of clinical practice guidelines which address treatment issues for alcohol and other drug problems. Addiction severity measures have also been developed to help guide treatment decisions. For example, the Addiction Severity Index (ASI) was developed by McLellan and his colleagues (1980). The ASI assesses seven areas, including medical, employment and legal status, use of alcohol or other drugs, family-social interactions, and psychiatric status. The ASI has been shown to be reliable and valid for measuring severity of addiction and for tracking improvement during treatment.

Alcoholics Anonymous (AA), probably the best known approach to alcohol addiction, is a common component of aftercare for many patients, and is believed by many to be highly effective for individuals who are motivated to follow its 12-step program. However, AA considers itself a "fellowship" rather than a treatment program, and there are no objective studies of its effectiveness for individuals who voluntarily participate. The AA model has been applied to other drugs with the formation of Narcotics Anonymous (NA) groups for people with problems with drugs other than alcohol. The only two controlled studies of AA, which were published many years ago (Brandsma et al., 1980; Ditman and Crawford, 1966), found no evidence that AA improved outcomes for participants who were *required* to attend AA meetings by the criminal justice system. Some controlled studies, although not specifically focused on AA, have included AA as one of the treatment groups. For example, a study by Walsh and colleagues (1991) randomly assigned 227 alcohol-dependent workers identified through employee assistance programs to one of three groups—compulsory inpatient treatment, compulsory AA attendance, or a choice of treatment option. This study found that the compulsory inpatient treatment group scored better than the other two groups on 12 job-performance and 12 drinking and drug-taking measures over a two-year period. Of the remainder, the group who chose their treatment scored better than the group assigned to compulsory AA attendance, a result especially pronounced among the workers who had used cocaine in addition to alcohol.

The Minnesota model of inpatient treatment is used for most alcohol inpatient treatment in the United States, but it has been largely evaluated in uncontrolled studies, making it difficult to determine its effectiveness (Hester, 1994; IOM, 1989). The only controlled study of the Minnesota model found that it was slightly more effective than a more traditional therapy-based inpatient approach used in Finland; no comparisons were made to other American treatment approaches or to a no-treatment control group (Keso and Salaspuro, 1990). The Minnesota model program typically has a standardized length of stay (usually 28 days) consisting of detoxification, followed by educational lectures on such topics as the disease concept of addiction, the effects of alcoholism (or drug abuse when applied to cocaine or other drugs) on families, relapse prevention techniques, and alternative coping mechanisms (Weiss, 1994). These programs often use self-disclosure forums similar to AA and NA and rely on group therapy and peer confrontation; recovering alcoholics often serve as counselors.

Chemical dependency treatment traditionally has been provided in an inpatient or residential program, although the term is increasingly used to refer to outpatient programs as well. In addition to the Minnesota Model, chemical dependency programs variously include 28-day, 12-step, or Hazelden-type treatment approaches, but these programs have traditionally been expensive and primarily for insured individuals (Gerstein, 1994). Chemical dependency programs were originally intended to treat alcohol problems, but they are now also used for patients who use illegal drugs. These programs usually provide intensive treatment, lasting 3 to 6 weeks, and patients help develop their own treatment plans patterned on the 12-step recovery model of AA and NA.

Therapeutic communities are considered another type of residential treatment, but include additional elements to address the multiple problems commonly associated with illegal drugs such as unemployment, criminal justice involvement, and other circumstances. Thus, these programs are important to consider for certain groups of individuals addicted to cocaine. Therapeutic communities provide treatment in a highly structured environment that typically uses no chemical agents except for medical or psychiatric reasons (Anglin and Hser, 1992). For individuals requiring extensive skills training and support in addition to drug treatment (e.g., homeless patients), therapeutic communities can be quite effective. These programs focus on the use of interpersonal relationships in an atmosphere of mutual self-help, and incorporate encounter group therapy, behavior modification, education classes, and residential job duties; later programs include jobs for clients who live in the facility and work in the outside community (De Leon, 1990; Sells, 1974). Treatment may be as short as 6 to 12 months, but traditional programs require at least 15 months in residence (Anglin and Hser, 1992). Phoenix House in New York City is a well-known example of a therapeutic community that treats all kinds of drug abuse.

National data from the Drug Abuse Reporting Project (DARP), collected from 1969 to 1973, and Treatment Outcomes Prospective Study (TOPS), collected between 1979 and 1981, studies indicated that therapeutic communities produced significant improvements in both immediate and long-term outcome (De Leon, 1984a,b). Drug use and criminal behavior decreased, while employment, school enrollment, and other pro-social behaviors increased (Anglin and Hser, 1992). A study at Phoenix House also showed increases in self-esteem and intelligence measures and decreases in personality disorders (De Leon, 1984b). Several studies indicated that clients who spent more time in therapeutic communities tended to improve more than those who spent less time (Anglin and Hser, 1992). Although high early drop-out rates were found to limit their effectiveness, individuals who managed to stay in the therapeutic community at least 12 months measurably benefited from the programs offered (De Leon, 1984b).

Certain important differences between treatment settings for alcohol or cocaine addiction need to be taken into account. For example, although studies have not demonstrated a clear advantage of initial inpatient treatment for alcoholism, in general there are greater medical complications from alcohol withdrawal than are observed from cocaine withdrawal (McLellan et al., 1997). Thus, inpatient treatment for alcoholism during the detoxification phase may be warranted for strictly medical reasons alone. Cocaine addiction can be initially treated taking an approach more focused on stabilization in an outpatient setting. One study comparing inpatient versus outpatient treatment for cocaine addiction found differences in completion of treatment between the groups, 89 percent completed inpatient versus 54 percent completed outpatient treatment, but a follow-up at 7 months revealed no differences between the groups in abstinence from cocaine (Alterman et al., 1994). This study however, excluded subjects with acute medical or psychiatric problems. It is known from many studies that drop-out rates are much higher among persons addicted to cocaine and, especially for those with significant co-occurring medical or psychiatric problems, inpatient treatment is likely to be more effective (Higgins et al., 1993; McLellan et al., 1997). Inpatient treatment may also be more useful for alcoholism if the patient has medical or psychiatric problems or is also abusing cocaine (Fleming and Barry, 1992), but may not be necessary in the absence of additional problems (Miller and Hester, 1986; Hayashida et al., 1989).

Psychosocial or Behavioral Therapies

The American Psychiatric Association (APA) guidelines for the treatment of addictive disorders involving alcohol, cocaine, and opioids (1995) were developed based on intensive literature reviews and input from many clinical and research experts. These guidelines recommend psychosocial treatment as an essential element of treatment for addiction. As with treatment setting, however, the specific type of therapy needed varies and must take into account a variety of patient factors. The APA guidelines specifically endorse therapies that address cognitive and behavioral approaches, psychodynamic and interpersonal therapies, group and family therapies, and participation in self-help groups (e.g., AA).

A well-known literature review of psychosocial and other treatments for alcohol problems conducted by Hester in 1994 identified several approaches that have "good evidence of effectiveness." These included behavioral marital therapy, brief interventions, community reinforcement approach, self-control training, social skills training, and stress management. These are described briefly below.

Behavioral marital therapy emphasizes improving communication and problem solving between spouses and increasing praise and other positive interactions.

Brief interventions, which may be provided by addiction specialists but are often provided by internists or other health care professionals in primary care settings, generally consist of the professional providing objective information about the patient's individual drinking problem, giving the patient the opportunity to take responsibility for changing his or her behavior, and one or two counseling sessions. These have been found in a number of studies to be as effective as longer-term inpatient and outpatient treatment (Bien et al., 1993; Hester, 1994; Kahan et al., 1995). It is important to note that these interventions often target at-risk individuals, do not necessarily result in total abstinence, and may vary in effectiveness in different populations (e.g., gender or different severity of drinking).

The **Community Reinforcement Approach** consists of a patient and therapist developing several strategies to address individual problems associated with alcohol abuse, such as taking Antabuse® (disulfiram), a drug that prevents drinking by causing an extremely unpleasant and potentially life-threatening physical reaction to alcohol; behavior-oriented marital counseling; and participation in healthy leisure time activities.

Self-control training teaches patients self-management skills that can be used to decrease or prevent alcohol consumption. These include setting goals, self-monitoring, rewarding oneself when goals are met, and learning new coping skills.

Social skills training teaches patients how to form and maintain interpersonal relationships.

Stress management teaches individuals relaxation strategies and other ways to reduce tension and manage stress.

Although more research has been done examining psychosocial treatments for alcohol addiction, recent studies indicate differences between various therapies in cocaine treatment. For example, one study compared cocaine-addicted patients randomly assigned to either behavioral counseling, based on the community reinforcement model, or drug abuse counseling, based on a disease model (Higgins et al., 1993). The study found that 58 percent of the patients in the behavioral counseling group completed the 24-week, outpatient treatment, compared to only 11 percent in the drug abuse counseling group. Further, at 8 weeks, 68 percent of the behavioral counseling group maintained complete abstinence from cocaine, compared to only 11 percent in the other group; at 16 weeks, 42 percent of the behavioral and 5 percent of the drug abuse group had maintained abstinence. Even with pharmacotherapy for depression, psychosocial therapy may provide added benefits according to a study in which patients were randomly assigned to one of four conditions: relapse prevention therapy (a cognitive behavioral approach) and antidepressant medication (desipramine); clinical management and antidepressant; relapse prevention and placebo; or clinical management and placebo (Carroll et al., 1994a). Although neither the psychosocial therapy nor pharmacotherapy condition was associated with treatment retention or reduction in cocaine use, the more intensive relapse prevention approach was associated with higher abstinence in patients with more severe addiction and greater responses to treatment by depressed patients. In a follow-up study at one year, this research group found that the effect of psychotherapy increased over time, producing a delayed, but significantly improved outcome (Carroll et al., 1994b).

Treating accompanying psychiatric symptoms with pharmacotherapy and other means also has been shown to be useful in alcoholism treatment. A randomized controlled trial found depressed patients treated with the antidepressant, desipramine, remained abstinent from alcohol longer than controls (Mason et al., 1996). Another study with actively drinking, depressed outpatients found a marked reduction in alcohol consumption (McGrath et al., 1996). Similarly, treatment of anxiety with buspirone resulted in longer retention, reduced anxiety, and fewer drinking days in anxious alcoholics (Kranzler et al., 1994).

Pharmacotherapy

As discussed previously, there are no replacement pharmacotherapies for alcoholism or cocaine addiction, but antidepressant, antianxiety, and other medications for accompanying psychiatric conditions are useful in the context of a comprehensive treatment program for addictive disorders involving alcohol and cocaine. A major advance in the treatment of alcoholism is the demonstrated efficacy of the opiate antagonist, naltrexone (ReVia™) in prolonging abstinence in alcoholism treatment. Naltrexone blocks opioid receptors in the brain reward system. When naltrexone was used in conjunction with behavioral therapy over a 3-month period, patients receiving the drug after discharge from inpatient treatment were half as likely to relapse compared to those receiving a placebo. Patients receiving naltrexone generally reported fewer drinking days, fewer drinks per session, and lowered craving scores (O'Malley et al., 1996). Naltrexone was approved by the Food and Drug Administration (FDA) for use in treating alcoholism in 1994, but it has not received enthusiastic support from many self-help groups, such as AA, many of whom believe that recovery from alcoholism is best accomplished by abstinence from all drugs.

In Europe two other drugs have been introduced for the treatment of alcohol addiction: acamprosate and gamma-hydroxybutyric acid. Studies have shown results with these medications similar to those seen with naltrexone (Gallimberti et al., 1992; Nalpas et al., 1990; Paille et al., 1995). For example, one randomized controlled trial found acamprosate resulted in higher early abstinence rates (67 percent at 60 days) compared to placebo (50 percent), longer abstinence duration (62 percent acamprosate, vs. 45 percent placebo), and lower drop-out rates (41 percent acamprosate, versus 60 percent placebo) (Sass et al., 1996). Both acamprosate and gamma-hydroxybutyric acid may mimic the actions of the neurotransmitter, gamma aminobutyric acid (GABA) in the brain, and additional clinical studies are underway in an effort to gain FDA approval for their use in the United States.

Disulfiram (Antabuse®) has been used for many years for the treatment of alcoholism. It causes nausea, vomiting, and other painful and potentially life-threatening side effects if alcohol is consumed, and must be taken daily, so its effectiveness depends on the patient's consistent compliance. Anton (1995) concluded that Disulfiram is effective when its use is closely monitored or where patients are highly motivated or very compliant. In recent years, innovative advanced behavior therapies have been used to sustain compliance.

Effective pharmacotherapy for cocaine addiction remains elusive and is a priority research issue, especially for the National Institute on Drug Abuse's (NIDA's) Medication Development Program (IOM, 1995a). Although pharmacotherapy for underlying psychiatric illness, such as the use of antidepressants to treat depression, seems to augment other therapeutic approaches in cocaine treatment, no medication has been found that specifically blocks craving for cocaine.

Matching Studies

Given the high number of variables that need to be considered in treatment of alcoholism or cocaine addiction, the research community has attempted to design studies to assess whether or not specific types of patients can be assigned to specific types of treatment to maximize the chances of success. This research, often referred to as patient-treatment matching, is aimed at providing an empirically derived knowledge base to improve patient placement criteria and treatment outcomes (McLellan and Alterman, 1991).

One of the largest of these studies, Project MATCH, was published in 1997 and involved an 8-year, multisite trial of alcoholism treatment that assessed three behavioral treatment conditions and 10 patient factors (NIAAA, 1997a). The treatment conditions were a 12-step facilitation therapy, cognitive-behavioral therapy (based on skill building to avoid relapse), and motivational enhancement therapy (based on using a patient's personal resources to effect change). The patient factors included alcoholism and psychiatric severity, cognitive and motivational, social support, and other types of measures. The results of this study were surprising and seemed to contradict clinical wisdom that the right "match" was necessary to optimize success. Of 11 hypothetical matches, only one was upheld by the data—patients with low psychiatric severity, treated as outpatients with 12-step facilitation therapy, did better than a similar group treated with cognitive-behavioral therapy. Interestingly, all participants in this study showed high levels of improvement, which were sustained over time, and one of the investigators has suggested that this improvement was the result of the overall high quality of treatment provided in the study across all treatment conditions (NIAAA, 1997b). If so, the study supports the concept that the overall quality of care across a range of treatment choices is crucial to the outcome of any given treatment.

It would be premature to conclude on the basis of the Project MATCH study that the concept of patient-treatment matching is flawed. One component not assessed in the study was pharmacotherapy, and future research will undoubtedly address more completely the effects of naltrexone in reducing craving for alcohol, as well as pharmacotherapies for co-occurring psychiatric conditions. There are already indications that such research will prove fruitful. For example, two recently published randomized trials studies suggest that treating depressed alcoholics with antidepressants and anxious alcoholics with anti-anxiety medications may be useful adjuncts to other treatment components (Kranzler et al., 1994; McGrath et al., 1996).

Multisite matching trials are underway to assess the effectiveness of different treatments for cocaine addiction, but individual studies offer support to the notion that attention to patient factors may be quite useful in determining treatment options for such patients. For example, the studies by Carroll and colleagues cited previously indicate that treating depression in cocaine-addicted patients with pharmacotherapy is associated with better outcomes and, thus, may be an appropriate match of multicomponent therapy with a specific patient characteristic (Carroll et al., 1994a,b).

TREATMENTS FOR OPIOID ADDICTION

Treatment for addiction to heroin and opioid drugs has many similarities to treatment for alcoholism or cocaine addiction. For example, the stages of treatment are the same, the same variety of types of treatment settings are used, and studies have examined the usefulness of a variety of treatment components. There is one clear difference and that is the availability of a "replacement" pharmacotherapy, methadone, for opioid addiction. Methadone substitutes for heroin but does not cause euphoria; thus, methadone can be used to help heroin-addicted individuals withdraw from heroin and avoid relapse. However, not all treatment strategies use methadone.

The four major types of publicly funded treatment programs for opioid addiction are detoxification, outpatient methadone maintenance, therapeutic communities, and outpatient drug-free programs (Anglin and Hser, 1992). Addiction research has tended to focus on the effectiveness of these publicly funded programs, especially for individuals addicted to heroin (see also Appendix E).

Another IOM committee has recommended replacing the term "detoxification" with "medically supervised withdrawal" to describe the acute or short-term (several days, several weeks, or a few months) administration of an approved long-acting opiate agonist drug to an individual patient, at a steadily reduced dose, on a schedule or rate such that the individual is able to continue to function with a tolerable level of discomfort and the use of short-acting opioids by the individual is discouraged (IOM, 1995b). However, research indicates that medically supervised withdrawal is relatively ineffective as a sole treatment. Many addicted individuals drop out of the programs as drug doses are progressively lowered (Lipton and Maranda, 1982; Maddux and Desmond, 1980), and the relapse rate is high; in one study 64 percent returned to daily opioid use during the first year, and 77 percent returned to some opioid use (Simpson and Sells, 1982). Many researchers and clinicians now consider a detoxification program to be an adjunct or precursor to other treatments rather than a treatment itself, since it can be used in emergency situations and enables addicted individuals to enter other treatment programs (McLellan et al., 1997).

Methadone Maintenance Pharmacotherapy

The IOM committee also recommended replacing the term "methadone maintenance" with "maintenance pharmacotherapy," which it defined as "sustained administration of an approved opiate agonist drug, at relatively stable doses, for the treatment of opiate addiction" (IOM, 1995b). Patients receive a stable dose, usually as outpatients, and are then usually required to receive counseling and rehabilitation services, undergo routine urine tests, and abstain from illegal opioid drugs. Maintenance pharmacotherapy is usually intended for patients who have been unable to succeed with drug-free forms of treatment (Anglin and Hser, 1992).

Maintenance pharmacotherapy has been extensively evaluated, and it has been found to significantly decrease opioid use and criminal behavior and improve general health while patients are in treatment, according to national data from DARP and TOPS, as well as other studies (Cooper et al., 1983; Senay, 1985; Tims and Ludford, 1984). After patients are taken off methadone, these improvements are still observable but lessen (Hser et al., 1988).

Researchers at UCLA who reviewed several studies reported that patients spent about 12 percent of their nonincarcerated time engaged in daily narcotics use while in methadone programs compared to about 70 percent when not in treatment, and the percentage of time that they abstained from all drugs increased from 12 percent to 26 percent (Anglin and Hser, 1992). Similarly, a study in New York City, Philadelphia, and Baltimore found that the average number of crime days per patient plunged from 307 days per year before treatment to 20 days per year after 6 months of treatment (Ball et al., 1987). In national experiments conducted after methadone programs closed, clients who did not enter other treatment programs were more likely to become readdicted to heroin, and their arrest and incarceration rates increased dramatically (Anglin and Hser, 1992).

New Pharmacotherapies for Opioid Addiction

Naltrexone (Revia™, formerly Trexan™), a selective opioid antagonist which was approved for the treatment of narcotic dependence in 1984, has been found to prevent relapse to opioid dependence in patients who are very highly motivated, such as parolees and health care professionals. This is the same dug that is also approved for use in treating alcoholism (see above). As an opioid antagonist, naltrexone works by preventing the euphoria and dependency-producing effects that would otherwise result from taking heroin or other opioid drugs.

As is generally the case for medical treatments of addiction, naltrexone has limited effectiveness when used alone and is significantly more effective in combination with behavior therapy or psychotherapy techniques (IOM, 1996).

These findings are consistent with the view that addiction is best understood and treated using several approaches, in this case combining psychological and pharmacological therapies (Anton et al., 1995).

LAAM (levo-alpha-acetylmethadol), a synthetic opioid, has been introduced in the United States for the treatment of opioid addiction under the trade name Orlaam® (see Appendix G). LAAM reduces euphoria and suppresses withdrawal symptoms for up to 72 hours (IOM, 1995a). It works like methadone, but requires only three doses weekly instead of daily dosing, thereby increasing compliance among those treated.

Buprenorphine is a partial opioid agonist that in clinical trials was effective in maintenance therapy and helped keep patients in treatment. Buprenorphine produces less physiological dependence than methadone, but it causes some euphoria and therefore can be abused. An oral form of buprenorphine, that is combined with naloxone to reduce the potential for abuse, is currently being tested. Naloxone is not absorbed orally, but it would block the euphoric effects of buprenorphine if someone injected the combined medication.

SMOKING CESSATION PROGRAMS

Much of this chapter has examined treatment for opioid or cocaine addiction and alcoholism. It is useful, however, to consider briefly the application of various treatment strategies for nicotine addiction. The vast majority of adult smokers have tried to quit or would like to quit. Most smokers who try to quit do so without any formal cessation program, and many are successful. However, smoking cessation clinics and self-help groups have proliferated to help smokers unable to quit on their own. Early clinics offered lectures, pamphlets, medication, and physician counseling (DHHS, 1991). Clinics were offered in most major cities and many smaller communities in the 1970s and 1980s; these included clinics conducted by nonprofit groups such as the American Cancer Society and the Seventh Day Adventist Church, and commercial programs such as SmokEnders. Regardless of the type of program used, many were effective in helping smokers abstain initially, but long-term quit rates tended to be low, even following advice from physicians to quit smoking (Ockene et al., 1991, 1994; Law and Tang, 1995). Nevertheless, many investigators have argued that even the small long-term results achieved through physician and dentist intervention are worth the effort and may be up to 17 times more effective than doing nothing (Sachs, 1990). Many of the programs and self-help groups have now incorporated newer techniques and educational materials about relapse prevention, and are increasingly viewed as one component of a variety of approaches to treat nicotine addiction.

In 1996, the Agency for Health Care Policy and Research (AHCPR) of DHHS issued guidelines to help physicians encourage patients to quit smoking.

The guidelines recommend that doctors ask every patient at every visit if they smoke; ask patients about their desire to quit smoking and reinforce such intentions, including helping set a quit date; motivate patients who are reluctant to quit; prescribe nicotine patches and nicotine gum; and refer patients for counseling when appropriate (DHHS, 1996).

Nicotine Chewing Gum

Nicotine chewing gum received FDA approval as an aid in smoking cessation in 1983 and was approved for over-the-counter use in 1996. The gum provides a slow release of nicotine, totaling 2 mg or 4 mg per piece (Haxby, 1995). Nicotine chewing gum has been thoroughly studied, and several meta-analyses clearly demonstrate its modest but statistically significant short-term effectiveness, especially when used in conjunction with intensive behavioral interventions (Cepeda-Benito, 1993; Haxby, 1995). Some studies indicate that nicotine gum is not effective when used with only brief advice and counseling in primary care settings; moreover, it is not effective in terms of long-term abstinence (Haxby, 1995); however, other studies suggest that nicotine gum can augment the effectiveness of brief physician interventions (Fiore et al., 1990; Ockene et al., 1991, 1994). There are several problems with the gum that may be responsible for its limited effectiveness. Perhaps most important, it has an unpleasant taste and 10 to 15 pieces must be chewed each day to provide the recommended nicotine replacement (Haxby, 1995). In addition, it requires a correct chewing technique and the avoidance of acidic beverages such as coffee, cola, and orange juice so that the nicotine is adequately absorbed (Haxby, 1995).

Nicotine Patches

Transdermal nicotine patches were approved by the FDA as smoking cessation aids in 1991 and 1992. Patches were first made available over-the-counter in 1996. Patches are easier to use than gum, because they deliver nicotine through the skin continuously over a 16- or 24-hour period. Despite skin reactions, which occur in 35 percent to 54 percent of patch users, compliance is considerably better than it is for the gum (Haxby, 1995). This greater compliance may account for the better success rates, which averaged twice as high as those using placebo patches (Fiore et al., 1992). Rates of smoking cessation varied greatly across studies, from a high of 77 percent 6 weeks after treatment to a low of only 18 percent three weeks after treatment (Fiore et al., 1992). Although success rates decrease after treatment is stopped, they are still considerably higher at 6 months than those for placebos, ranging from 22 percent to 42 percent compared to 2 percent to 28 percent for placebo patches (Fiore et al., 1992).

Only recently has the combined use of nicotine patches and nicotine gum in overcoming nicotine addiction begun to be studied. By adding nicotine gum use, active patch users supplement their sustained nicotine release from the patch with repeated increases of plasma nicotine concentrations from the gum, helping to reduce withdrawal symptoms associated with abstinence from smoking (Benowitz, 1993; Fagerström, 1994; Fagerström et al., 1993). A preliminary study suggests that adding nicotine gum use to active patch use can increase abstinence rates among people who smoke 10 cigarettes or more a day—a statistically significant increase up to 6 months (Kornitzer et al., 1995). For those who used both the patch and gum, the abstinence rate was 27 percent after 6 months and 18 percent after 1 year (Kornitzer et al., 1995).

Studies similar to investigations with cocaine and alcohol are underway to assess the usefulness of antidepressant and other pharmacotherapies in addition to nicotine replacement. For example, the use of naltrexone is under investigation to reduce craving. Such studies have shown sufficient evidence of effectiveness of the antidepressant, bupropion hydrochloride (Wellbutrin®), for the FDA to approve its use, in May 1997, in conjunction with nicotine gum or patches, for treating nicotine addiction. All of the replacement and pharmacotherapeutic strategies for nicotine addiction are recommended to be used in conjunction with behavioral interventions, such as participation in support groups.

CONCLUSION

Extensive research has shown that treatment for addiction is as effective as treatments for other chronic, relapsing medical conditions. Advances in pharmacotherapy (Appendix G), basic science (Appendix F), and behavioral and social science research (Appendix H) have allowed the development of useful multimodal therapies for addiction that combine pharmacological and behavioral approaches. There are nevertheless significant differences in the treatment of specific addictions (e.g., cocaine versus opioid) and the challenge for future research is to identify ways to improve treatment success across a variety of conditions. Table 5.2 lists some of the key challenges to be addressed, requiring ongoing research in a variety of disciplines and a better base of interdisciplinary and health services and treatment outcomes research.

TABLE 5.2 Some Future Challenges in Pharmacotherapy and Treatment Research

General Issues

- Development of better conceptual approaches to treatment evaluation
- Development of models of optimal pharmacological and behavioral interactions
- Evaluation of cue-dependent craving and clinical approaches to minimize the likelihood of relapse
- Development of objective measurements of craving in humans and development of animal models of craving
- Determination of the long-term (longer than 1 year) efficacy of brief intervention strategies and examination of factors predictive of success—for example, gender differences.
- Exploration of combination pharmacotherapy—for example, opioid antagonist and serotonin reuptake inhibitors in treating alcoholism relapse and craving. This approach appears reasonable in view of the multisite influence of ethanol in the regulation of the mesolimbic dopamine pathway by opioids, 5-HT and GABA. Further determination of subsets of alcoholics who might be more responsive to pharmacotherapy should be made
- Examination of the relationship between alcohol abuse and the abuse of cocaine, nicotine, opioids, and other drugs
- Examination of the behavioral consequences of the interaction of alcohol with other drugs of abuse and evaluation of the effect of medications for the treatment of codependence problems

Nicotine

- Evaluation of optimal combination of pharmacotherapy (with one drug or multiple drugs) and behavioral intervention for relapse prevention in humans
- Development of an acceptable nicotine antagonist for motivated smokers who have not succeeded with nicotine replacement therapy
- Further development of patient-treatment matching, especially treatments targeted at those subpopulations where smoking is most prevalent (e.g., smoking and alcohol, smoking and use of other psychoactive drugs, smoking in chronic psychotic patients)

Opioids

- Evaluation of optimal combination of pharmacotherapy (with one drug or multiple drugs) and behavioral intervention for relapse prevention in humans
- Demonstration of effectiveness of opioid tolerance and dependence blocking drugs in humans

Stimulants

- Evaluation of optimal combination of pharmacotherapy (with one drug or multiple drugs) and behavioral intervention for relapse prevention in humans
- Successful demonstration of cocaine antagonist or partial agonist drugs in blocking cocaine effects in humans

TABLE 5.2 Continued

Alcohol

• Evaluation of optimal combination of pharmacotherapy (with one drug or multiple drugs) and behavioral intervention for relapse prevention in humans

• Establishment of better physiological markers of alcohol use and risk of alcoholism in humans

---

REFERENCES

Alterman AI, O'Brien CP, McLellan AT, August DS, Snider EC, Dobra M, Cornish JW, Hall CP, Raphaelson AH, Schrade FX. 1994. Effectiveness and costs of inpatient versus day hospital cocaine rehabilitation. *Journal of Nervous and Mental Diseases* 182(3):157–163.

American Psychiatric Association. 1995. *Practice Guidelines for the Treatment of Patients with Substance Abuse Disorders: Alcohol, Cocaine, Opioids.* Washington, DC: American Psychiatric Association.

American Society of Addiction Medicine. 1997. *Patient Placement Criteria for the Treatment of Substance-Related Disorders.* Second Edition. Washington, DC: American Society of Addiction Medicine.

Anglin D, Hser Y-I. 1992. Treatment of drug abuse. In: Watson RW, ed. *Drug Abuse Treatment. Drug and Alcohol Abuse Research.* Vol. 3. New York: Humana Press. Pp. 393–460.

Anton RF. 1995. Commentary: Disulfiram treatment of alcoholism. *Alcohol Health and Research World* 19(1):56–57.

Anton RF, Kranzler HR, Meyer RE. 1995. Neurobehavioral aspects of pharmacotherapy of alcohol dependence. *Clinical Neuroscience* 3:145–155.

Ball JC, Corty E, Bond H, Myers C, Tommasello A. 1987. The Reduction of Intravenous Heroin Use, Non-Opioid Abuse and Crime during Methadone Maintenance Treatment—Further Findings. In: Harris LS, ed. *Problems of Drug Dependence, 1987.* NIDA Research Monograph 81. Rockville, MD: National Institute on Drug Abuse. Pp. 224–230.

Benowitz NL. 1993. Nicotine replacement therapy. What has been accomplished—Can we do better? *Drugs* 45:157–170.

Bien TH, Miller WR, Tonigan JS. 1993. Brief interventions for alcohol problems. A review. *Addiction* 88:315–336.

Brandsma JM, Maultsby MC, Welsh RJ. 1980. *The Outpatient Treatment of Alcoholism: A Review and Comparative Study.* Baltimore: University Park Press.

Carroll KM, Rounsaville BJ, Gordon LT, Nich C, Jatlow P, Bisighini RM, Gawin FH. 1994a. Psychotherapy and pharmacotherapy for ambulatory cocaine abusers. *Archives of General Psychiatry* 51(3):177–187.

Carroll KM, Rounsaville BJ, Nich C, Gordon LT, Wirtz PW, Gawin F. 1994b. One-year follow-up of psychotherapy and pharmacotherapy for cocaine dependence. Delayed emergence of psychotherapy effects. *Archives of General Psychiatry* 51(12):989–997.

Cepeda-Benito A. 1993. Meta-analytical review of the efficacy of nicotine chewing gum in smoking treatment programs. *Journal of Consulting and Clinical Psychology* 61(5):822–830.

Cooper JR, Altman F, Brown BS, Czechowicz D, eds. 1983. *Research on the Treatment of Narcotics Addiction: State of the Art*. NIDA Research Monograph. DHHS Publication No. (ADM) 83-1281. Rockville, MD: National Institute on Drug Abuse.

De Leon G. 1984a. Program-based evaluation research in therapeutic communities. In: Tims FM, Ludford JP, eds. *Drug Abuse Treatment Evaluations: Strategies, Process, and Prospects*. NIDA Research Monograph 51. Rockville, MD: National Institute on Drug Abuse. Pp. 69–87.

De Leon G. 1984b. *The Therapeutic Community: Study of Effectiveness*. NIDA Research Monograph Series. DHHS Publication No. (ADM) 84-1286. Rockville, MD: National Institute on Drug Abuse.

De Leon G. 1990. The therapeutic community and behavioral science. *The International Journal of the Addictions* 25(12A):1537–1557.

DHHS (U.S. Department of Health and Human Services). 1991. *Strategies to Control Tobacco Use in the United States: A Blueprint for Public Health Action in the 1990s*. Smoking and Tobacco Control Monographs 1. Rockville, MD: National Cancer Institute, U.S. Department of Health and Human Services. October.

DHHS. 1996. *FDA Tobacco Regulation: Proposed Rule and Final Regulation*. Press Release. Washington, DC: Press Office, U.S. Department of Health and Human Services.

Ditman KS, Crawford GG. 1966. The use of court probation in the management of the alcohol addict. *American Journal of Psychiatry* 122:757–762.

Fagerström KO. 1994. Combined use of nicotine replacement products. *Health Values* 18:15–20.

Fagerström KO, Schneider NG, Lunell E. 1993. Effectiveness of nicotine patch and nicotine gum as individual versus combined treatments for tobacco withdrawal symptoms. *Psychopharmacology* 111:271–277.

Fiore MC, Pierce JP, Remington PL, Fiore BJ. 1990. Cigarette cessation: The clinician's role in cessation, prevention, and public health. *Disease-a-Month* 36(4):181–242.

Fiore MC, Jorenby DE, Baker TB, Kenford SL. 1992. Tobacco dependence and the nicotine patch. *Journal of the American Medical Association* 268(19):2687–2694.

Flemming MF, Barry KL, eds. 1992. *Addictive Disorders*. St. Louis:Mosby Yearbook Primary Care Series.

Gallimberti L, Ferri M, Ferrara SD, Fadda F, Gessa GL. 1992. Gamma-hydroxybutyric acid in the treatment of alcohol dependence: A double-blind study. *Alcohol: Clinical and Experimental Research* 16(4):673–676.

Gerstein DR. 1994. Outcome research: Drug abuse. In: Galanter M, Kleber HD, eds. *Textbook of Substance Abuse Treatment*. Washington, DC: American Psychiatric Press, Inc. Pp. 45–64.

Haxby DG. 1995. Treatment of nicotine dependence. *American Journal of Health-System Pharmacists* 52:265–281.

Hayashida M, Alterman AI, McLellan AT, O'Brien CP, Purtill JJ, Volpicelli JR, Raphaelson AH, Hall CP. 1989. Comparative effectiveness of inpatient and outpatient detoxification in patients with mild-to-moderate alcohol withdrawal syndrome. *The New England Journal of Medicine* 320(6):358–365.

Hester RK. 1994. Outcome research: Alcoholism. In: Galanter M, Kleber HD, eds. *Textbook of Substance Abuse Treatment.* Washington, DC: American Psychiatric Press, Inc. Pp. 35–43.

Higgins ST, Budney AJ, Bickel WK, Hughes JR, Badger G. 1993. Achieving cocaine abstinence with a behavioral approach. *American Journal of Psychiatry* 150(5):763–769.

Hser Y-I, Anglin MD, Chou C. 1988. Evaluation of drug abuse treatment: A repeated measure design assessing methadone maintenance. *Evaluation Review* 12(5):547–570.

IOM (Institute of Medicine). 1989. *Prevention and Treatment of Alcohol Problems: Research Opportunities.* Washington, DC: National Academy Press.

IOM. 1995a. *The Development of Medications for the Treatment of Opioid and Cocaine Addictions: Issues for the Government and Private Sector.* Washington, DC: National Academy Press.

IOM. 1995b. *Federal Regulation of Methadone Treatment.* Washington, DC: National Academy Press.

IOM. 1996. *Pathways of Addiction: Opportunities in Drug Abuse Research.* Washington, DC: National Academy Press.

Kahan M, Wilson L, Becker L. 1995. Effectiveness of physician-based interventions with problem drinkers: A review. *Canadian Medical Association Journal* 152(6):851–859.

Keso L, Salaspuro M. 1990. Inpatient treatment of employed alcoholics: A randomized clinical trial on Hazelden-type and traditional treatment. *Alcohol: Clinical and Experimental Research* 14:584–589.

Kornitzer M, Boutsen M, Dramaix M, Thijs J, Gustavsson G. 1995. Combined use of nicotine patch and gum in smoking cessation: A placebo-controlled clinical trial. *Preventive Medicine* 24:41–47.

Kranzler HR, Burleson JA, Del Boca FK, Babor TF, Korner P, Brown J, Bohn MJ. 1994. Buspirone treatment of anxious alcoholics. A placebo-controlled trial. *Archives of General Psychiatry* 51(9):720–731.

Law M, Tang JL. 1995. An analysis of the effectiveness of interventions intended to help people stop smoking. *Archives of Internal Medicine* 155(18):1933–1941.

Lipton DS, Maranda MJ. 1982. Detoxification from heroin dependency: An overview of methods and effectiveness. *Advances in Alcohol and Substance Abuse* 2:31–55.

Maddux JF, Desmond DP. 1980. Outpatient methadone withdrawal for heroin dependence. *American Journal of Drug and Alcohol Abuse* 7(3/4):323–333.

Mason BJ, Kocsis JH, Ritvo EC, Cutler RB. 1996. A double-blind, placebo-controlled trial of desipramine for primary alcohol dependence stratified on the presence or absence of major depression. *Journal of the American Medical Association* 275(10):761–767.

McGrath PJ, Nunes EV, Stewart JW, Goldman D, Agosti V, Ocepek-Welikson K, Quitkin FM. 1996. Imipramine treatment of alcoholics with primary depression: A placebo-controlled clinical trial. *Archives of General Psychiatry* 53(3):232–240.

McLellan AT, Alterman AI. 1991. Patient treatment matching: A conceptual and methodological review with suggestions for future research. In: Pickens RW, Leukefeld CG, Shuster CR, eds. *Improving Drug Treatment.* Research Monograph 106. Washington, DC: National Institute on Drug Abuse.

McLellan AT, Bender M, McKay JR, Zanis D, Alterman AI. 1997. Can the outcomes research literature inform the search for quality indicators in substance abuse treatment? In:. *Managing Managed Care: Quality Improvement in Behavioral Health.* Washington, DC: National Academy Press.

McLellan AT, Luborsky L, O'Brien CP, Woody GE. 1980. An improved evaluation instrument for substance abuse patients: The Addiction Severity Index. *Journal of Nervous and Mental Diseases* 168:26–33.

McLellan AT, Metzger DS, Alterman AI, Woody GE, Durrell J, Weisner CW, O'Brien CP. 1995. Is treatment for substance dependence "worth it?": Public health expectations, policy-based comparisons. *Training About Alcohol and Substance Abuse for All Primary Care Physicians.* Proceedings of a conference sponsored by the Josiah Macy, Jr. Foundation. New York.

Miller WR, Hester RK. 1986. Inpatient alcoholism treatment: Who benefits? *American Psychologist* 41:794–805.

Nalpas B, Dabadie H, Parot P, Paccalin J. 1990. L'acamprosate. De la pharmacologie a la clinique. *Encephale* 16(3):175–179.

NIAAA (National Institute on Alcohol Abuse and Alcoholism). 1997a. Matching alcoholism treatments to client heterogeneity: Project MATCH posttreatment drinking outcomes. *Journal of Studies on Alcohol* 58(1):7–29.

NIAAA. 1997b. NIAAA Reports Project MATCH Main Findings [WWW Document]. URL http://www.niaaa.nih.gov/events/match.htm (accessed March 7, 1997).

O'Brien CP, McLellan AT. 1996. Myths about the treatment of addiction. *Lancet* 347:237–240.

Ockene JK, Kristeller J, Goldberg R, Amick TL, Pekow PS, Hosmer D, Quirk M, Kalan K. 1991. Increasing the efficiency of physician-delivered smoking interventions: A randomized clinical trial. *Journal of General Internal Medicine* 6(1):1–8.

Ockene JK, Kristeller J, Pbert L, Herbert JR, Luippold R, Goldberg RJ, Landon J, Kalan K. 1994. The physician-delivered smoking intervention project: Can short-term interventions produce long-term effects for a general outpatient population? *Health Psychology* 13(3):278–281.

O'Malley SS, Jaffe AJ, Chang G, Rode S, Schottenfeld R, Meyer RE, Rounsaville B. 1996. Six-month follow-up of naltrexone and psychotherapy for alcohol dependence. *Archives of General Psychiatry* 53:217–224.

Paille FM, Guelfi JD, Perkins AC, Royer RJ, Steru L, Parot P. 1995. Double-blind randomized multicentre trial of acamprosate in maintaining abstinence from alcohol. *Alcohol and Alcoholism* 30(2):239–247.

Sachs DP. 1990. Smoking cessation strategies: What works, what doesn't. *Journal of the American Dental Association* Suppl:13S–19S.

Sass H, Soyka M, Mann K, Zieglgansberger W. 1996. Relapse prevention by acamprosate. Results from a placebo-controlled study on alcohol dependence. *Archives of General Psychiatry* 53(8):673–680.

Sells SB, ed. 1974. *Evaluation of Treatment.* Vols. 1 and 2. Cambridge, MA: Ballinger.

Senay EC. 1985. Methadone maintenance treatment. *The International Journal of the Addictions* 20(6–7):803–821.

Simpson DD, Sells SB. 1982. Effectiveness of treatment for drug abuse: An overview of the DARP research program. *Advances in Alcohol and Substance Abuse* 2(1):7–29.

Tims FM, Ludford JP, eds. 1984. *Drug Abuse Treatment Evaluation: Strategies, Progress, and Prospects.* NIDA Research Monograph 51. Rockville, MD: National Institute on Drug Abuse.

Walsh DC, Hingson RW, Merrigan DM, Levenson SM, Cupples LA, Heeran T, Coffman GA, Becker CA, Barker TA, Hamilton SK, et al. 1991. A randomized trial of treatment options for alcohol-abusing workers. *The New England Journal of Medicine* 325(11): 775–782.

Weiss RD. 1994. Inpatient treatment. In: Galanter M, Kleber HD, eds. *Textbook of Substance Abuse Treatment.* Washington, DC: American Psychiatric Press, Inc. Pp. 359–368.

6

Education and Training

Addiction research poses an exciting challenge for young scientists who wish to address one of the most important and persistent problems confronting society today (see Chapter 2). However, a number of factors may present obstacles to talented researchers considering a career in addiction research. One often-cited obstacle is the lack of the educational and training opportunities necessary to attract and support students and young professionals—and to encourage them to stay in the field during periods in which opportunities in other fields seem more attractive.

Based on the workshop and quantitative information collected during the study, the committee identified obstacles in both research and public arenas that may deter young investigators from entering addiction research. Obstacles within the research arena include lack of educational and training opportunities, lack of opportunities for integrative and collaborative research, and lack of adequate and stable funding (see Preface). This chapter focuses mainly on the educational and training opportunities in secondary schools, undergraduate institutions, and graduate and professional schools, as well as issues specific to research training and support during the early career years. Chapter 7 addresses the resource issues for new professionals in the field, and Chapter 8 addresses the obstacles presented in the public arena.

CAREER PATHWAYS

Career pathways for scientists and physician researchers are varied and present numerous points at which decisions can be made regarding career alternatives (NRC, 1994). As is the case for many careers that require graduate degrees, an interest in addiction research is likely to develop in college or graduate/medical school. However, the decision-making process starts much earlier; unless teenagers are already interested in scientific or medical careers, they are unlikely to take the undergraduate courses that could expose them to information about addiction or prepare them for graduate or professional school programs that train addiction researchers.

Some undergraduate students will seek particular graduate programs because they have already decided that they want to learn more about addiction or pursue a career in addiction research. Others will be interested in related research issues and come into contact with patients, faculty, course work, or research projects that encourage them to specialize in the field of drug abuse and addiction.

Until 15 years ago, most basic, clinical, and behavioral researchers in drug addiction received their doctoral training in pharmacology, experimental psychology, or a social science field. More recently, doctoral training programs in neuroscience have been established in many academic institutions; students in these programs have the kinds of interests and educational backgrounds that are particularly compatible with a career in addiction research. Recent addiction-related developments in the areas of biology and molecular genetics, cell and developmental biology, neurobiology, immunology, and behavioral pharmacology present compelling biological questions which are also attracting new investigators into the field of addiction research. M.D. and M.D./Ph.D. students also may become interested in treating addicted persons or be drawn to the theories and research on addiction. Several programs for such students, funded by the federal government, the private sector, or other institutions, provide integrated research and clinical experiences relevant to addiction.

Many students and young investigators, however, are not exposed to addiction research during their undergraduate, graduate, or medical school training because there are relatively few addiction-related courses offered at colleges, universities, and medical schools. Responses to the IOM survey from university and medical school administrators suggest that there is a lack of commitment on the part of many academic institutions to teach the subject area and formidable barriers to adopting new educational curricula which include more training and education about addictive disease.[1] These include competition with other subjects, the perception by many faculty members that the area is not scientifically

---

[1]The committee sent a questionnaire to 13 undergraduate, graduate, and medical schools inquiring about educational opportunities and barriers related to drug abuse and alcoholism for students. The results summarized are based on the responses (personal communication) from the questionnaires.

important, and the limited number of adequately trained faculty to teach such courses.

SECONDARY SCHOOL AND UNDERGRADUATE EDUCATION

All secondary schools offer science courses and many offer classes in psychology, sociology, or health education. Scientific information about drug addiction should be integrated into all these courses in high schools, colleges, and vocational schools. In addition, any classes or programs aimed at discouraging drug use should include factual, scientific information on the nature of drug abuse and should communicate that scientists are engaged in ongoing research in preventing and treating addiction.

Strategies are needed to enhance the educational curricula in drug addiction so that students learn about the genetic and biological bases for addiction and how they interact with psychosocial and behavioral factors in the development of addiction, efforts to overcome it, and relapse. There is also the complementary need to improve the expertise of faculty, so that well-qualified professionals who are capable of developing the necessary curricula are available to teach students about addicted individuals and addiction research.

Organizations such as the American Association for the Advancement of Science (AAAS) and the Faculty for Undergraduate Neuroscience (FUN) are attempting to broaden scientific knowledge at the K–12 and undergraduate levels, respectively (see Boxes 6.1 and 6.2). Such programs should include addiction research in their curricula.

Teenagers are exposed to a wide range of role models in various careers, but they are unlikely to know any addiction researchers, or even to read about them or see them on television. However, if there were more addiction researchers at colleges and universities, undergraduate students would be more likely to be inspired by their work and consider careers in the field. In addition and consistent with goals to increase the number of minorities and women in science and medicine, special attention should be paid to identifying women and minorities as role models.

Recommendations

To enhance interest in drug abuse research and foster a more complete understanding of the causes and consequences of drug abuse in secondary and undergraduate programs, the committee recommends:

• **The U.S. Department of Education should provide incentives for schools to increase emphasis on the physiological and psychosocial aspects of drug abuse and addiction in science and health education classes at elementary, middle school, and high school levels; and**

BOX 6.1
American Association for the Advancement of Science

The American Association for the Advancement of Science (AAAS) is a non-profit professional society dedicated to the advancement of scientific and technological excellence across all disciplines and to the public's understanding of science and technology. AAAS pursues a number of activities with implications for raising the profile of substance abuse research, a few of which are listed below.

Project 2061. A long-term initiative to reform K–12 education so that all high school graduates are science literate. The project produced *Science for All Americans* in 1989, which outlines what all students should be able to do in science, mathematics, and technology areas by the end of the K–12 period. In 1993, *Benchmarks for Science Literacy*, a curriculum design tool, was published. The report set knowledge goals for students completing grades 2, 5, 8, and 12. An upcoming computer resource called *Designs for Science Literacy* will help educators analyze their own science literacy and analyze curriculum elements to determine which elements help to achieve science literacy goals. Ultimately, the project will produce a comprehensive computer-based design for construction of a K–12 curriculum.

Science + Literacy for Health. This project, supported by the National Institute on Drug Abuse (NIDA), combines adult literacy efforts with science literacy and health information. The effort will target low-reading-level adults in literacy programs and community-based substance abuse and mental health education programs. The project has produced two books relevant to raising the profile of drug abuse: *The Brain Book* which covers brain function and injury, tumors, strokes, and Alzheimer's and Parkinson's diseases; and *Brain and Behavior,* which covers how the brain and behavior can be affected by mental disorders and drug abuse. Finally, AAAS recently received funding from NIDA to develop a drug education curriculum to be used by adult literacy and family literacy educators through a three-year project called the *Science + Literacy for Health Drug Education Partnership.*

SOURCE: AAAS (1996).

• Professional societies should facilitate expanding coverage of a science-based approach to understanding drug abuse and addiction at the university undergraduate level, especially in general psychology, sociology, and biology courses. Additional reviews should also be undertaken of related curricula in departments of social work, rehabilitation, and health education.

Box 6.2
Faculty for Undergraduate Neuroscience

The Faculty for Undergraduate Neuroscience (FUN) was established in 1991 to represent the concerns of neuroscientists teaching at undergraduate colleges and universities. FUN is an offshoot of the Society of Neuroscience and maintains close links with the parent organization. The group seeks to broaden knowledge and training in science, particularly the critical exposure to original research undertakings that may be absent from the traditional "prepackaged" curriculum experience. According to its 1993 mission statement, FUN is pursuing five goals:

1. the establishment of a Travel Award to support travel to Society for Neuroscience annual meetings by outstanding undergraduate neuroscience students.
2. the establishment of a Society for Neuroscience Award for Excellence in Undergraduate Teaching.
3. the establishment of a Travel Award for faculty from institutions with no travel support.
4. the creation of a newsletter highlighting undergraduate teaching.
5. the development of a mechanism for supporting regional faculty development workshops for neuroscience faculty from primarily undergraduate colleges and universities.

SOURCE: FUN (1996).

GRADUATE AND PROFESSIONAL EDUCATION

Curricula

Graduate School Programs

Graduate schools offer relatively few courses in substance abuse, a situation that has not changed over the last two decades. For example, in 1978–1979, Selin and Svanum (1981) conducted a survey of clinical psychology programs that were approved by the American Psychological Association (APA) and found that students received only minimal training in drug use and abuse. Lubin and his colleagues replicated the study in 1984, including APA-approved counseling psychology programs as well as clinical psychology programs, and found that there were no discernible differences in the quantity or quality of courses compared to the 1978–1979 results (Lubin et al., 1986). The study was again replicated in 1991–1992, adding APA-approved professional psychology (PsyD) programs in clinical psychology to the PhD clinical programs, but excluding counseling programs (Chiert et al., 1994). Once again, the authors found no differences compared to the earlier studies.

These surveys, which were completed by between 79 and 82 programs each time, indicated that very few faculty had expertise in substance abuse, and most schools did not offer any courses in the subject. For example, the estimated number of faculty with interests in "alcoholism/ substance abuse" ranged from 7 percent in 1978–1979 to 10 percent in 1991–1992. The number of schools offering at least one graduate-level course ranged from 42 percent in 1978–1979 to 38 percent in 1991–1992, but all but one of these courses were elective.

The 1991–1992 survey asked questions about specialization that had not been asked in the earlier surveys. Interestingly, it found that 52 percent of the schools offered practicum placements in institutions dealing primarily with substance abuse, and 76 percent indicated at least one current research project in the area (Chiert et al., 1994).

No data are available on the number of sociology departments with courses on addiction, although the American Sociological Association (ASA) reports that eight graduate programs offer specialty concentrations in substance abuse (ASA, 1996).

Graduate programs in pharmacy also have shortcomings, but efforts are underway to improve their curricula in the area of addiction. In the late 1980s, a survey of pharmacy faculty found that two-thirds believe their curriculum is inadequate in the area of drug and alcohol abuse. In 1988, the board of directors of the American Association of Colleges of Pharmacy adopted guidelines for curriculum development in drug and alcohol abuse (Baldwin et al., 1991).

It appears that there are more opportunities for training in drug abuse counseling than in research-oriented programs, and these opportunities are primarily at a less advanced educational level. The National Association of Alcoholism and Drug Abuse Counselors (NAADAC) lists 44 programs that offer graduate or postgraduate degrees, 38 that offer bachelor's degrees, and 77 that offer associate degrees (NAADAC, 1996).

These examples indicate that courses in addiction are not widely available on most university campuses. The lack of drug addiction research curricula at the undergraduate and graduate school level may discourage students who are interested in the field.

Medical School Programs

The lack of rigorous instruction on drug abuse and addiction is a particular problem in medical schools. Less than 1 percent of curriculum time is spent on drug addiction studies in U.S. medical schools (Durfee et al., 1994); few programs devote more than a few hours of class time to the topic within required or elective courses. Furthermore, only four of 121 medical schools reported requiring a separate course on alcohol and drug abuse (AAMC, 1997), and specific curricula have not been widely adopted (Durfee et al., 1994), as they have by many specialties (e.g., pharmacology) (Baldwin et al., 1991), psychiatry (Halikas, 1992), primary care and family medicine (Davis et al., 1992, 1993), and pediatrics (Kokotailo et al., 1995). In addition, courses on addiction may be offered in several different departments (IOM, 1995) and their overlapping or inconsistent content may discourage students from taking more than one.

A concerted effort to stimulate medical school education in addiction medicine began in 1972 with the Career Teacher program sponsored by NIAAA and NIDA. The program, which is no longer funded, originally trained faculty to develop and implement curricula; it was funded in 59 U.S. medical schools. Currently, the U.S. Center for Substance Abuse Prevention (CSAP) sponsors a faculty development program, begun in 1989, which funds programs in 34 schools of medicine, nursing, social work, and psychology (IOM, 1995).

Only two medical schools have curricula and programs on drug addiction that are cited by those in the field as models: Harvard Medical School and the University of Pennsylvania School of Medicine (see Boxes 6.3 and 6.4). Harvard's four-year-old program includes required courses and course elements in the first two years and then various elective rotations, basic science seminars, and senior clinical electives. The program includes 60–70 faculty members whose primary focus is drug abuse issues. The University of Pennsylvania School of Medicine drug abuse curriculum, established in 1990, provides a basic introduction to addiction issues through lectures and elective rotations. Most of the course work is in the psychiatry department, and there are 10–15 faculty members involved.

In other medical schools, the number of required and elective courses has increased in recent years, but the number of faculty with expertise in addiction who are available to teach these courses or serve as mentors is low compared to those with expertise in other chronic diseases (Durfee et al., 1994; Kokotailo et al., 1995). A rigorous, systematic evaluation of those curricula and the specific educational needs of medical students and of health professions in other specialties has not been conducted, nor has there been any systematic evaluation of training programs. Because such evaluations can be quite expensive consideration needs to be given to a variety of less costly strategies to improve coverage of these topics in medical schools.

Reflecting the lack of attention to addiction as part of medical school curricula, many educational institutions and even accreditation boards tend to ignore the issues of addiction completely. For example, there are few questions on drug addiction on the national medical and board specialty examinations (Chappel and Lewis, 1992; Schnoll et al., 1993). The lack of emphasis on this health and social issue is likely to convey a message to young professionals that is not important.

BOX 6.3
Case Study: Harvard Medical School, Division on Addictions

This 4-year-old program for addiction medicine focuses on required courses and course elements in years one and two, and various elective rotations, basic science seminars, and senior clinical electives in years three and four.

Faculty: Approximately 360 affiliated faculty members (60–70 with a primary focus on substance abuse issues).

Educational Task Force: Approximately 20 faculty from the 7 teaching hospitals affiliated with Harvard University. The group is charged with evaluation of course content ensuring sufficient depth and breadth.

Program Evaluation: A recent evaluation found several problems. These included findings that medical students (1) do not view successes; (2) are not taught to recognize substance abuse in an inpatient setting; (3) do not learn to make appropriate referrals; and (4) do not have good role models.

Barriers: Several barriers to improving the situation were identified: (1) lack of knowledge; (2) stigma and prejudice; (3) social acceptance of some drugs (i.e., alcohol and nicotine); (4) physician addiction; (5) denial (by physician and/or patient); and (6) enabling by the physician (e.g., overprescribing).

Potential Solutions: Several improvements were suggested: (1) expose students to patients with successful outcomes; (2) address physician addiction; (3) faculty development (better mentors); (4) increase patient exposure during first two years of curriculum.

Student Feedback: In the fall of 1993, two medical students who saw gaps in their substance abuse training proposed a project to correct the problem. The result was a collaboration by 38 medical students and 16 faculty on the *Source Book on Substance Abuse and Addiction* (Friedman et al., 1995).

Community Involvement Project: The medical school's Division on Addictions is developing, in cooperation with the community of Billerica, Massachusetts and the Merrimack Valley Educational Collaborative, an addiction science curriculum. The goal is to improve basic science education in grades 6–12 by using the scientific method and focusing on substance abuse and addiction science as examples.

SOURCE: Thurmond (1995–1996).

Finally, clinical experiences are an essential part of the medical school curriculum, and exposure to addiction issues in clinical settings could be an important influence on medical students' career decisions. However, intentional exposure to addicts and addiction issues does not happen often during graduate training or medical residency. As one young investigator stated, "Perhaps if more residents had mandatory training in addiction treatment, the field would be more likely to be considered important and interesting" (IOM, 1996).

BOX 6.4
Case Study: University of Pennsylvania, School of Medicine

The substance abuse curriculum at the University of Pennsylvania School of Medicine and Veterans Affairs Medical Center was established in 1990 as a result of the periodic curriculum review process, including a student-faculty retreat. The program provides a basic introduction to substance abuse through selected lectures and elective rotations. The bulk of the course work is in the psychiatry department.

Faculty: Approximately 10–15 affiliated faculty members (most with psychiatry training and an added qualification in addiction medicine).

Barriers to Improving Curriculum: The major barriers are (1) competition for time in an already crowded curriculum; (2) ambivalence about the study of substance abuse or belief held by some faculty that it is less important; and (3) a persistent perception problem—is addiction a disease or simply bad behavior?

Clinical Research Fellowship in Substance Abuse: A highlight of the substance abuse program is the clinical research fellowship program, run by the Department of Psychiatry and Veterans Affairs Medical Center's Treatment Research Center. The two-year fellowship program provides mostly clinical and some basic research training for physicians and postdoctoral fellows in the treatment of substance abusers. All fellows participate in clinical rotations, but focus their research in one of several laboratories affiliated with the program.

Training Program: All program participants are assigned a mentor with whom they meet weekly. The first year of the program consists mostly of clinical rotations supplemented by course work focusing on research methodology and ethics and biostatistics, particularly in the substance abuse field. During the second year, fellows engage in full-time research and publicly present the findings. Participants are also guided through the process of writing a NIDA/NIH-style grant application before the end of the program.

SOURCE: Cancro (1996); O'Brien (1996); Woody (1996).

Strategies

Increasing course work and clinical experience in addictive disorders would have benefits beyond the recruitment of new physician-scientists into the field. For one thing, approximately half of all medical students and residents will become primary care providers. Thus, improving the curricula and enhancing exposure to addiction during clinical training would increase medical students' knowledge and awareness and positive attitudes and beliefs and help them better identify drug abuse and addiction problems (Gopalan et al., 1992).

Multidisciplinary teaching addressing medical, epidemiological, public health, behavioral, and social science perspectives on drug addiction should be incorporated into mainstream educational curricula for all medical students and many other health professionals. In addition, specialty board examinations should include questions on drug addiction. Finally, because students need to be properly prepared to work in a clinical environment and have an understanding of the clinical needs of this field and the approaches to treatment, opportunities to work in clinical settings should be incorporated into medical training.

An innovative program to improve physicians' ability to diagnose and treat addiction has been established by the North Carolina Governor's Institute on Alcohol and Substance Abuse, Inc. In 1992, the Kate B. Reynolds Charitable Trust Fund provided $887,479 to the Governor's Institute to help promote curricula changes in the state's medical schools. The goal of the changes was to better equip medical students with the necessary skills and knowledge to prevent addiction and identify, intervene with, and manage addicted individuals. Evaluation of the institute's modification of curricula at four medical schools (Duke University, University of North Carolina, Bowman Gray at Wake Forest University, and East Carolina University) related to alcohol and drug abuse found that the amount of alcohol and drug abuse education increased, educational materials and activities related to alcohol and drugs were developed, greater interaction occurred in teaching and research across disciplines and departments, familiarity with the curriculum development process increased, and faculty development programs were initiated and enhanced (North Carolina Governor's Institute, 1996a). The Governor's Institute also works closely with universities to provide seed money for young investigators in addiction research (see Box 6.5). The committee believes that strategies similar to the North Carolina program should be encouraged.

Recommendations

Although there are many opportunities in educational and training programs for addiction researchers, serious gaps remain that can reduce the knowledge, ability, and potential impact of those treating addictive disorders. An effective educational and training system must be responsive to the different needs associated with individuals at various stages of their careers and in different disciplines. Continuity and early exposure are integral elements in such a system (see Appendix I).

BOX 6.5
North Carolina Governor's Institute on
Alcohol and Substance Abuse, Inc.

Goals: The institute seeks to bring about concerted action to strengthen curricula and pioneer new training methods for both students and professionals through interaction with drug abuse research and treatment programs. A related and mutually supportive goal is to aid communication among all health professionals, especially those working in primary care settings and drug abuse treatment programs.

Structure and Role: The institute is a private, nonprofit organization created in 1990 to address the special needs of health professionals for better education and more information about the complex social and medical problems of substance use, misuse, abuse, and dependency. The institute works with university medical centers; community hospitals and treatment facilities; Area Health Education Centers (AHEC); state and local public health and mental health agencies; federal agencies, such as the Center for Substance Abuse Treatment, NIDA, and NIAAA; and professional organizations including medical, dental, nursing, social work, clinical psychology, pharmacy, and drug abuse professionals. The institute acts as a catalyst and broker to promote cooperative action.

Scholarship Programs: *The Young Investigator Award Program in Biomedical/Substance Abuse Research.* The program, established in 1993, is a statewide, peer-reviewed award funded by the Burroughs Wellcome Fund. Its goal is to identify and promote the development of scientists who will perform research into the causes and effects of drug abuse with the goal of improving treatment modalities. The program provides one year of start-up funding of $5,000 to $12,000 for projects that can later be supported by outside sources. Each young investigator presents his or her findings at the following year's institute annual statewide conference. Applicants must be in an accredited postdoctoral educational program or in the first 48 months of a faculty appointment at a university in North Carolina. In its first three years, the program funded 12 of 37 applicants.

Public Policy Scholars Program. This program, established in 1992, is funded by the North Carolina Division of Mental Health, Developmental Disabilities, and Substance Abuse Services. The program seeks to stimulate graduate students' and health professionals' interest in drug abuse and to produce information that will lead to a better understanding of drug abuse. The program awards support short-term research studies on drug abuse issues and their health and public policy implications. In 1995–1996 10 awardees will receive $2,500 each; they must present their findings in a televised public forum. Applicants must be graduate or medical students, postdoctoral fellows, or medical residents in North Carolina academic health sciences programs. In its first three years, the program funded 33 of 65 applicants.

continues on next page

BOX 6.5 Continued

Other Activities:
- statewide multidisciplinary conferences on current issues;
- drug abuse curriculum development in the four medical schools and one dental school in North Carolina;
- basic skills track for clinicians at the North Carolina School for Alcohol and Drug Studies;
- survey of regulatory problems involved in prescription drug misuse, abuse, and diversion;
- inventory of nursing education on drug abuse;
- development of a database and linkages with other drug abuse databases; and
- furnishing speakers for AHEC programs.

SOURCE: North Carolina Governor's Institute (1996b,c,d).

The committee recommends that:

- **Accreditation and certifying entities [e.g., Liaison Committee on Medical Education (LCME), American Psychological Association (APA)] should review curricula in medical schools and in psychology, social work, and nursing departments for the adequacy of drug addiction courses and should require basic competence in these areas for certification and recertification on medical specialty board examinations and in other relevant disciplines;**
- **Deans, administrators, and professional societies should undertake systematic evaluation of existing curricula to assess how they encourage or discourage training in addiction research and develop curricula tailored to different levels of schooling and specialty. Incentives should be provided to recruit and train faculty to teach courses in addiction research and to serve as role models.**

THE IMPORTANCE OF MENTORS

Exposure to course work and clinical experiences in the area of addiction is a potentially important way to generate students' interest in addiction research careers. In addition, as in all areas of medicine, some investigators are motivated by personal reasons, such as having family members or friends with drug abuse or addiction problems. However, most of the new investigators who attended the committee's workshop highlighted the importance of their mentors and role models in their career decisions.

The lack of courses in addiction starts a cycle of shortages at every stage of the pipeline for professionals in the field of addiction research: fewer undergraduates are exposed to scientific information about addiction, so that fewer graduate students and medical students express interest in the field; thus administrators do not seek faculty who are experts in the field, resulting in fewer young professionals on the faculty, and, ultimately, fewer senior faculty. A cause and an effect of these shortages is a lack of mentors at many institutions.

Undergraduates are influenced by the role models they meet in college and in their communities during a trial-and-error learning process which occurs early in their formative university years. A mentor, by contrast, is more actively engaged with a student but unlikely to be an important influence until graduate or professional school. Given the apparent importance of mentors for young investigators currently in the field, the shortage of faculty who have expertise in drug addiction and can serve as mentors is a serious problem (Chappel, 1991). At the March 1996 IOM workshop, several new investigators reported that good mentors were difficult or impossible to find in the schools (IOM, 1996). In addition, they noted the lack of female and minority role models. Several young investigators expressed the belief that research and treatment in the field tend to be dominated by males and that female students would benefit from female role models especially in dealing with patients who are difficult or threatening.

It is well known that clinical supervision provides the most effective means for improving clinical skills (Chappel and Lewis, 1992). Clinical researchers depend upon experienced role models and mentors to build a solid foundation in understanding and treating patients. However, the committee found that the lack of mentors was a particular problem for clinical addiction researchers. There was also some evidence of an insufficient number of qualified researchers in the behavioral and social sciences to serve as role models for graduate students interested in pursuing addiction research, particularly in combination with the M.D. degree. For example, the behavioral and social sciences are excluded from the Medical Sciences Training Program (MSTP), which provides federal funding to pursue M.D./Ph.D. degrees jointly.

Although there is empirical literature concerning the importance of mentoring on shaping careers, relatively little of this research has been conducted in the fields of medicine or addiction research. A study of psychiatry faculty at 116 medical schools found that M.D.s listed faculty and other mentors as most influential in their decision to obtain research training; those trained in Ph.D. and M.D./Ph.D. programs cited faculty and other mentors as the second most influential factors in their decisions to become trained as researchers (Pincus et al., 1995). The central role of mentors is further underscored by the finding that time spent with a mentor was seen as an integral part of a research training program and provided guidance into specified areas of research and career development (Pincus et al., 1995).

Strategies to Enhance the Role of Mentors

Mentors are needed at all stages of research training as well as for different groups of students, such as women and minorities. There is no single strategy for increasing and sustaining the number and quality of mentors; several different efforts are needed.

One strategy would be to make more attractive existing programs provide mentorship opportunities for students. The Senior Scientist Award (K05) and the Academic Career Award (K07), offered to both the junior and senior researcher levels,[2] could include mentoring qualifications to support this development. These and other awards should be further encouraged and reviewed to ensure that they are attracting the most capable mentors and that the awards are closely coupled with the mentored career development awards for biomedical and behavioral scientists. For example, NIDA and NIAAA in the past jointly sponsored a Career Teacher Training Program—which was cut from the budget during the Reagan years—and placed career teachers in nearly 60 medical schools (Pokorny and Solomon, 1983). These and other programs would be particularly useful if available at the research centers that offer the best training environments in terms of breadth and depth for emerging scientists.

The committee believes there is a critical need for mentors trained in interdisciplinary approaches. The committee supports the development of new pre- and postdoctoral fellowships that provide comprehensive and intensive training in sound research methods and practical research experience in drug addiction, using mentoring by an interdisciplinary group (two or more) of experienced investigators.

Another strategy would be to develop a network of mentors to provide opportunities for co-mentoring when the available mentors at the young investigator's department or institution lack critical expertise in areas required to conduct a particular research project. In those instances, the young investigator would have a mentor on-site but would obtain additional technical assistance from another person who might be located at a different institution. To facilitate geographically remote mentoring relationships, satellite mentoring programs could be established through the network of mentors. To gain a better understanding

---

[2]Following a recent evaluation of the 19 career award grants (K grants) for new, senior, and clinical scientists, NIH reduced the number to 6 categories and clarified the career development goals of each. The new K awards (K01, K02, K05, K07, K08, K12) offer institutes more flexibility to target and train new investigators and expand the careers of those already in the field. The K07 award is used to support individuals interested in introducing or improving curricula, at the junior level with guidance from a mentor, and at the senior level to improve curricula and enhance the research capacity within an academic institution, thus increasing the visibility and overall support of the field. Over the past several years, NIDA adopted a strategy that increased the number of mentored career development awards (i.e., K01 and K08) from 5 in FY 1991 to 53 in FY 1995.

of the role of mentors in various research career pathways (i.e., neurological, clinical, and behavioral), it would help to assess systematically the effects of various aspects of mentoring experiences on subsequent research involvement. Strategies aimed at providing staggered intervals of mentoring at various stages of training might also be useful, for example, short-term internships to expose researchers in addiction to the clinical setting or educational materials that yield an accurate picture of the clinical experience. Incentives for such exposure could be provided through joint programs with industry, foundations, universities, and government.

Ways to overcome the unique difficulties in designing and conducting addiction research are best learned from good mentoring relationships, where students learn by example how to work with, manage, test, and treat some extremely difficult patients. Mentors in a clinical setting can help develop suitable and testable hypotheses, critique papers, assure that adequate research time is available for collecting pilot data, and assist with grant applications. Clinical mentors are also important to help address some of the problems, such as lack of time, competing demands, and financial support, that lead to the high attrition rates in addiction research by health professionals.

Recommendations

To promote appropriate mentoring, the committee recommends that:

- **Ph.D. programs in the behavioral and social sciences should be included among the degrees eligible for M.D./Ph.D. (MSTP) support;**
- **NIDA and NIAAA should increase the number of mentors by promoting interdisciplinary research through the establishment of funding mechanisms for mentoring teams composed of investigators from different disciplines in the Academic Centers of Excellence programs;**
- **NIDA and NIAAA should emphasize innovative mentoring programs through the K05, K07, and other K award mechanisms; and**
- **NIDA and NIAAA should consider reviving the Career Teacher Training Program.**

SPECIALIZATION AND CREDENTIALING ISSUES

Although the focus of this report is on addiction *research*, the issues of treatment and research are often intertwined. Faculty with expertise in treating drug-addicted individuals can stimulate faculty who have expertise in conducting basic or applied research on addiction. Likewise, the availability and quality of *treatment* are dependent on innovative research findings. Furthermore, many graduate students, medical students, postdoctoral students, and medical residents will be exposed to the field of addiction research while being supervised in treatment settings.

Professionals who deal with the public concerning mental health and drug addiction need to be familiar with the scientific research regarding addiction (Chapters 3, 4, and 5). Currently, many professionals do not possess the information they need to inform others. If the goal is to ensure appropriate and effective treatment and research, drug addiction must be taught as part of the educational credentialing process of all health care providers, and there should be rigorous standards for specialization as well. One way to achieve this would be better translation of research into treatment, particularly community-based treatment programs and providers, and better use of clinical experience in the design of research studies. This topic is the concern of another IOM committee, the Committee on Community-Based Drug Treatment, whose report is expected in 1998.

Overall, the committee found limited opportunities for credentialing, specialization, and accreditation for the practice of drug abuse treatment. Strategies are needed to encourage wider adoption of a credentialing process for addiction across the range of medical and health care specialties.

Board certification has become an important postdoctoral licensing mechanism for physicians in the United States (Moore and Lang, 1981). Many hospitals and managed care organizations require board certification in a physician's field of specialty (IOM, 1995). In the addiction field, there has been some pressure for physician certification from third-party insurance carriers and regulatory agencies to establish the qualifications of physicians responsible for drug treatment (Chappel and Lewis, 1992).

In some specialty areas there has been positive movement toward certification opportunities. In 1991, the American Board of Psychiatry and Neurology (ABPN), in concurrence with the American Board of Medical Specialties, officially established the field of addiction psychiatry as an area of subspecialization. Board certification of psychiatrists involved in addiction treatment provides a means of identifying properly trained and experienced addiction psychiatrists. Similarly, APA recently established a College of Professional Psychology to certify licensed psychologists in proficiency areas of practice; the first program established criteria for a certification program in alcohol and drug abuse. Although other professional associations have not followed suit, the American Society of Addiction Medicine (ASAM) has established certification examinations for its members and continues to request the American Medical Association (AMA) to ask each of the primary care specialties' certifying boards to study the desirability and feasibility of offering subspecialty examinations in addiction medicine (ASAM, 1997).

Although addiction medicine may not become a board-certified specialty, most professional associations and organizations provide and recommend continuing medical education (CME) courses in drug addiction. For example, the Association for Medical Education and Research in Substance Abuse

(AMERSA) promotes postgraduate medical education on drug addiction through curriculum development and national meetings.

Recommendations

The committee recommends that:

- All treatment professionals should have some knowledge of basic neuroscience and how alcohol, nicotine, and other drugs work on brain pathways, influence behavior, and interact with diverse conditions. Treatment professionals should include physicians, nurses, clinical psychologists, social workers, drug abuse peer counselors, and other health care providers who work in conjunction with one another in treating patients with an addictive disease;
- Continuing education courses to update treatment professionals' knowledge base on addiction should be instituted systematically and widely; and
- Competence-based documentation of treatment professionals' knowledge base on addiction should be sought in licensing and recertification examinations.

CONCLUSION

A number of strategies are necessary to attract talented students into the field of addiction research. Incorporation of additional information about the process of addiction in precollege and undergraduate science classes, for example, may not only interest young people planning a research or medical career but it can also increase public understanding of addiction. The challenge in graduate and medical school programs is to increase the amount of information presented in a variety of ways, including course work, clinical experiences, research fellowship opportunities, and other mechanisms. Throughout the educational experience, however, mentors and role models provide often critical input in the career decisions of talented young people. Thus, ways to develop and enhance teachers and mentors with expertise in addiction research would be very useful long-term strategies. Finally, increased attention to addiction in medical specialty board examinations and other professional certification programs is needed to foster a greater understanding of addiction by professionals leading eventually to integration of the diagnosis and treatment of addiction into general medical and primary health care settings.

REFERENCES

AAAS (American Association for the Advancement of Science). 1996. *The American Association for the Advancement of Science World Wide Web Homepage.* [http://www.aaas.org]. October.

AAMC (Association of American Medical Colleges). 1997. *Curriculum Directory 1996–1997.* 25th Edition. Washington, DC: Association of American Medical Colleges.

ASA (American Sociological Association). 1996. Personal communication to the Institute of Medicine. September.

ASAM (American Society of Addiction Medicine). 1997. *Training as Prerequisite to Recognition of Sub-specialization in Addiction Medicine—Resolution A-97.* Submitted to the American Medical Association.

Baldwin J, Light K, Srock C, Ives T, Crabtree B, Miederhoff P, Tommasello T, Levein P. 1991. Curricula guidelines for pharmacy education: Substance abuse and addictive disease. *American Journal of Pharmaceutical Education* 55:311–316.

Cancro MP. 1996. Personal communication to the Institute of Medicine. Spring.

Chappel JN. 1991. Educational approaches to prescribing practices and substance abuse. *Journal of Psychoactive Drugs* 23:359–363.

Chappel JN, Lewis D. 1992. Medical education in substance abuse. In: Lowinson JH, Ruiz P, Millman RB, eds. *Substance Abuse: A Comprehensive Textbook.* 2nd Edition. Baltimore: Williams & Wilkins. Pp. 958–969.

Chiert T, Gold SN, Taylor J. 1994. Substance abuse training in APA-accredited doctoral programs in clinical psychology: A survey. *Professional Psychology: Research and Practice* 25(1):80–84.

Davis AK, Graham A, Coggan P, Finch J, Fleming M, Brown R, Sherwood R, Henry R, Schulz J. 1992. Creating a substance abuse network in family medicine: Lessons learned. *Family Medicine* 24:299–302.

Davis A, Parran T, Graham A. 1993. Educational strategies for clinicians. *Primary Care* 20:241–250.

Durfee M, Warren D, Sdao-Jarvie K. 1994. A model for answering the substance abuse educational needs of health professionals: The North Carolina Governor's Institute on Alcohol and Substance Abuse. *Alcohol* 11(6):483–487.

Friedman L, Fleming NF, Roberts DH, Hyman S. 1995. *Source Book on Substance Abuse and Addiction.* Baltimore: Williams & Wilkins.

FUN (Faculty for Undergraduate Neuroscience). 1996. *The Faculty for Undergraduate Neuroscience World Wide Web Homepage.* [http://cvax.ipfw.indiana.edu/~wilsonj/fun.htm]. October.

Gopalan R, Santora P, Stokes E, Moore R, Levine D. 1992. Evaluation of a model curriculum on substance abuse at The Johns Hopkins University School of Medicine. *Academic Medicine* 67:261–266.

Halikas J. 1992. Model curriculum for alcohol and drug abuse training and experience during the adult psychiatry residency. *American Academy of Psychiatrists in Alcoholism and Addictions* 1:222–228.

IOM (Institute of Medicine). 1995. *The Development of Medications for the Treatment of Opiate and Cocaine Addictions.* Washington, DC: National Academy Press.

IOM. 1996. *Workshop on Identifying Strategies to Raise the Profile of Substance Abuse and Alcoholism Research.* Washington, DC: Committee to Identify Strategies to Raise the Profile of Substance Abuse and Alcoholism Research. March 28–29.

Kokotailo P, Fleming M, Koscik R. 1995. A model alcohol and other drug use curriculum for pediatric residents. *Academic Medicine* 70:495–498.

Lubin B, Brady K, Woodward L, Thomas EA. 1986. Graduate professional psychology training in alcoholism and substance abuse: 1984. *Professional Psychology: Research and Practice* 17(2):151–154.

Moore FD, Lang SM. 1981. Board-certified physicians in the United States. *The New England Journal of Medicine* 304:1078–1084.

NAADAC (National Association of Alcoholism and Drug Abuse Counselors). 1996. *National Association of Alcoholism and Drug Abuse Counselors Education and Research Foundation: List of Educational Opportunities in the Alcoholism and Drug Abuse Counseling Field.* [http://www.csic.com/edu/index.html]. October.

North Carolina Governor's Institute on Alcohol and Substance Abuse, Inc. 1996a. *Draft Report: Final Report to Kate B. Reynolds Charitable Trust Fund.* Research Triangle Park, NC: North Carolina Governor's Institute on Alcohol and Substance Abuse, Inc.

North Carolina Governor's Institute on Alcohol and Substance Abuse, Inc. 1996b. *Fact Sheet.* Research Triangle Park, NC: North Carolina Governor's Institute on Alcohol and Substance Abuse, Inc.

North Carolina Governor's Institute on Alcohol and Substance Abuse, Inc. 1996c. *Public Policy Scholars Program 1995–1996: Call for Proposals.* Research Triangle Park, NC: North Carolina Governor's Institute on Alcohol and Substance Abuse, Inc.

North Carolina Governor's Institute on Alcohol and Substance Abuse, Inc. 1996d. *Young Investigator Award Program in Biomedical/Substance Abuse Research.* Research Triangle Park, NC: North Carolina Governor's Institute on Alcohol and Substance Abuse, Inc.

NRC (National Research Council). 1994. *The Funding of Young Investigators in the Biological and Biomedical Sciences.* Washington, DC: National Academy Press.

O'Brien CP. 1996. Personal communication to the Institute of Medicine. January.

Pincus HA, Haviland MG, Dial TH, Hendryx MS. 1995. The relationship of postdoctoral research training to current research activities of faculty in academic departments of psychiatry. *The American Journal of Psychiatry* 152(4):596–601.

Pokorny AD and Solomon J. 1983. A Follow-Up Survey of Drug Abuse and Alcoholism Teaching in Medical Schools. *Journal of Medical Education* 58:316–321.

Schnoll S, Durburg J, Griffin J, Gitlow S, Hunter RB, Sack J, Stimmel B, deWit H, Jara GB. 1993. Physician certification in addiction medicine 1986–1990: A four-year experience. *Journal of Addictive Diseases* 12(1):123–133.

Selin JO, Svanum S. 1981. Alcoholism and substance abuse training: A survey of graduate programs in clinical psychology. *Professional Psychology* 12:717–721.

Thurmond CH. 1995–1996. Personal communication to the Institute of Medicine. December–February.

7

Resources Needed for Young Investigators

This chapter briefly examines the funding structures and levels for advanced training in addiction research in the context of more general pressures confronting young investigators. In addition, the chapter explores some special problems for clinical researchers, particularly physician scientists, and outlines some examples of nonfederal funding strategies. Recommendations directed toward a variety of agencies and foundations are made in this chapter.

Young investigators trained in the disciplines relevant to addiction research seek postdoctoral fellowships or salaried positions in universities, academic medical centers, or pharmaceutical companies. Those who seek academic careers usually apply for positions where the salary is at least partly secure, but their ability to conduct research is often dependent on research funding that has been obtained by a colleague (such as a senior researcher in charge of the postdoctoral training program) or funding that they must obtain by writing or helping to write a successful research grant application. The launching of a research career or the sustained development of a career thus depends upon the availability of fellowship programs, research grants, and other mechanisms.

The effectiveness of individual fellowships, institutional traineeships, grant-funded research assistantships, and other programs is currently under review by both the National Institutes of Health (NIH) and the National Science Foundation (NSF) (Mervis, 1996). Large national surveys, however, rarely identify trends specific to addiction research. Thus, it is useful to examine the funding streams specific to this area of research in the context of the overall funding structure for postgraduate training.

Federally supported research career paths often include efforts to obtain the National Research Service Awards (NRSA) predoctoral and postdoctoral training fellowships (e.g., T32, F31, F32), followed by career development awards (e.g., K01, K02, K08, etc.), and general research grant funding mechanisms (e.g., R29, R01, R37). These are available through NIH; two institutes, the National Institute on Drug Abuse (NIDA) and the National Institute on Alcohol Abuse and Alcoholism (NIAAA), use these awards for addiction researchers. Each program has its own set of requirements, duration of support, and funding (see Box 7.1).

BOX 7.1
Description of Awards

F30 *(Individual Predoctoral National Research Service Awards for M.D./Ph.D. Fellowships)*—The fellowship provides support for both medical school and predoctoral Ph.D. training. The maximum duration is 6 years (4 years if being used to cover tuition). A stipend of $10,008 is provided to cover living expenses.

F31 *(Individual Predoctoral National Research Service Awards for Fellows)*—The fellowship award provides up to 5 years' support for predoctoral students enrolled in a doctoral degree program. A stipend of $10,008 to cover living expenses is included. The fellowship also requires that the awardee work with an approved mentor or sponsor actively doing research in the area.

F32 *(Individual Postdoctoral National Research Service Awards for Fellows)*—The award provides up to 3 years of aggregate support for scientists who have completed a degree with the goal of broadening their background or extending their research potential. In FY 1994, the average NIH F32 was $24,500 with the duration depending on the number of years of relevant postdoctoral experience possessed by the candidate. Awardees must pursue their research training on a full-time basis (40 hours/week) with research clinicians confining clinical duties within the training experience. Furthermore, fellows incur a service obligation of 1 month for each month of support in the first 12 months of postdoctoral NSRA support.

T32 *(National Research Service Award Institutional Research Training Grant)*—The grant provides up to 5 years of renewable support to institutions for various levels of training, including predoctoral research training, postdoctoral research training, clinical research training, and short-term research training for health professional students.

T35 *(National Research Service Award Short-Term Institutional Research Training Grant)*—The grant provides support to institutions offering research training opportunities to individuals or students during off-quarters or summers to continue or initiate their research experience. The positions should last longer than 2 but less than 3 months.

K01 *(Mentored Research Scientist Development Award)*—The award provides 3 to 5 years of support for an intensive, supervised career development experience in one of the biomedical, behavioral, or clinical sciences. The program should focus on novel or highly promising multidisciplinary approaches to the problem. The applicant must identify an experienced mentor willing to provide 75 percent support for the duration of the award.

K02 *(Independent Scientist Award)*—This award provides up to 5 years of support for newly independent scientists who can demonstrate the need for a period of intensive research focus as a means of enhancing their research careers. The applicant must have a doctoral degree and peer-reviewed, independent, research support at the time the award is made and be willing to spend at least 75 percent time on research and research career development.

K05 *(Senior Scientist Award)*—The 5-year award provides stability of support to outstanding scientists who have demonstrated a sustained, high level of productivity and whose expertise, research accomplishments, and contributions to the field have been and will continue to be critical to the mission of the particular NIH center or institute. The candidate must have long-term support from an institute or center and peer-reviewed grant support at the time of the award.

K07 *(Academic Career Award)*—The award is used to provide support for individuals interested in introducing or improving curriculum in a particular scientific field as a means of improving the educational or research capacity at the grantee institution. The support may be of two types: (1) leadership—a 5-year award for more senior individuals; and (2) development—a 2- to 5-year mentored award for more junior candidates. Candidates for the leadership award must be willing to devote at least 25 percent effort to the program and development candidates 75 percent time.

K08 *(Mentored Clinical Scientist Development Award)*—The 3- to 5-year award supports the development of outstanding clinician research scientists through a period of supervised research experience that may integrate didactic studies with laboratory or clinically based research. The applicant must have a clinical degree or equivalent, have initiated postgraduate clinical training, and be willing to devote at least 75 percent effort to the program.

R01 *(Research Project)*—Research project grants are awarded to institutions on behalf of a principal investigator to facilitate pursuit of a scientific focus objective. Institutional sponsorship assures NIH that the institution will provide facilities and be accountable for the grant funds.

continues on next page

BOX 7.1 Continued

R03 *(Small Grant)*—The awards provide research support, specifically limited in time and amount, for various activities such as pilot projects, testing of new techniques, or feasibility studies of innovative, high-risk research, which would provide a basis for more extended research.

R21 *(Exploratory/Developmental Grant)*—A small, limited time award to encourage the development of new research activities in categorical program areas.

R29 *(First Independent Research Support and Transition [FIRST] Award)*—The award is designed to assist newly independent researchers. The award, usually for 5 years, provides an opportunity for a research scientist who has completed training to become an independent investigator.

R37 *(Method to Extend Research in Time [MERIT] Award)*—The award provides long-term grant support to investigators whose research competence and productivity are distinctly superior and who are highly likely to continue to perform in an outstanding manner. Investigators may not apply for a MERIT award. Program staff and/or members of the cognizant National Advisory Council/Board will identify candidates for the award during review of competing research grant applications.

SOURCE: NIH (1996c).

At the committee's workshop, new investigators and senior investigators expressed their perceptions that obtaining initial research funding from NIDA and NIAAA is difficult because of the instability of these funds and the competition for them. To assess the accuracy of these perceptions, the committee examined trends in overall funding, the number of applications and awards, and application success rates for the various mechanisms. Comparative data across several institutes are shown to provide a useful context for understanding the career development issues involved in addiction research. Information is provided for NIDA, NIAAA, the National Institute of Mental Health (NIMH), the National Cancer Institute (NCI), and the National Heart, Lung, and Blood Institute (NHLBI). The latter were selected because they represent chronic and prevalent medical diseases (see Chapter 2 and Table 7.1 for a discussion of the comparative costs to society for cancer, mental disorders, and other chronic diseases).

TABLE 7.1 Total Costs to Society and NIH Training and Research Support for Specific Diseases (millions of dollars)

Disease	Year	Total Costs[a] to Society	1995 Research Budget	1995 Training Budget	Training Budget Percent of Research Budget
Drug Addiction[b]	1990	$256,800	$472.1	$14.5	3.1
Cancer (all sites)[c]	1990	96,100	1,215.5	38.6	3.2
Heart Diseases[c]	1991	125,800	982.6	48.0	4.9
Mental Disorders	1990	147,800	454.2	30.9	6.8

NOTE: Research and training figures taken from budgets of related NIH institutes (i.e., drug addiction: NIDA, NIAAA; cancer: NCI; heart diseases: NHLBI; mental disorders: NIMH). 1990 is used as the base year because it is the most recent date for which the total costs to society of substance addiction and mental disorders have been estimated. For comparison, total cost estimates for cancer and heart diseases are based on the years listed closest to 1990. However, given that the cost estimates were calculated by different sources, the numbers may not be directly comparable and serve only to provide an overview of the estimated cost of each illness to society.

[a]Includes direct and indirect costs.
[b]Total for alcohol, illicit drugs, and nicotine (includes costs of AIDS and fetal alcohol syndrome).
[c]Includes costs of adverse health effects of drugs, particularly nicotine.

SOURCE: IOM (1995), NHLBI (1994), NIH (1996a, 1997), Rice (1995), Varmus (1995), and see Table 2.3.

FUNDING LEVELS

Total institute budgets, research grant budgets, and training grant budgets for the past 10 years are shown in Figures 7.1 through 7.3. Although there have been increases in total budgets in actual dollars, when inflation is taken into consideration the growth has been more limited, except for NCI and NIDA.[1] Since FY 1990, research grant budgets have increased between 18 percent to 30 percent, with NIDA increasing by 24 percent and NIAAA by 21 percent. Although training budgets show a different trend—in the direction of convergence for NIDA and NIAAA with the other three institutes—both NIDA's and

[1]It is important to note that many graduate students and post-doctoral fellows are also supported on research grants.

NIAAA's training budgets are significantly lower than the others when measured as the percentage of training dollars to total research dollars.

THE PIPELINE

Comparative data on the total numbers of applicants and awardees for training and fellowship awards (T32, F31, and F32) and for career development research awards (R29 and R01) show that there are fewer investigators at all stages of the pipeline for both NIDA and NIAAA than for the other institutes (Figures 7.4 through 7.7). In fact, between 1975 and 1992 only a small proportion (3 percent) of the National Research Service Awards (NRSA) trainees and fellows were supported by NIAAA (327 individuals) and NIDA (310 individuals). In recent years, the number of awards for traineeships and fellowships has been increasing overall for both NIDA and NIAAA, but they are still far fewer than at the other three institutes (Pion, 1996). There has been considerable growth over the past 10 years in the number of applicants for NIDA and NIAAA career development awards (R29 and R01). The number of awards doubled for NIDA, but has fluctuated rather than consistently increased for NIAAA.

Vulnerable Junctures and Lack of Research Training

Investigators at early stages of their research careers frequently progress from an extended period of postdoctoral research training support to the First Independent Research Support and Transition (FIRST) award (i.e., R29 support). This 5-year award is designed to provide an opportunity for a research scientist who has completed training to become an independent investigator. The committee learned, however, that this is a particularly vulnerable time, making attrition from the pipeline a serious problem at this juncture. Many of the young investigators at the workshop expressed concern about this difficult transition and the low prospects for receiving support. Because of the reduced number of available tenure track positions in many fields, young investigators are increasingly finding themselves in postdoctoral positions or nontenure track, semi-dependent positions for extended periods of time. There is increased concern that there are few permanent jobs available following completion of postdoctoral training fellowships. Some junior and senior investigators stated that they had chosen to leave the field, or research altogether, as a result in part of their frustration about obtaining subsequent career development awards. The vulnerability during this interval is considerable, however, for all young investigators. The delay between training fellowship and career development grant for NIAAA has increased from less than 1.4 years before FY 1990 to just less than 3 years in 1995; for NIH in general the increase has been from 1.7 to 2.4 years.

A second point of vulnerability in the pipeline is the R01 award, which is a research project grant awarded to institutions on behalf of a principal investigator. Although data demonstrate that investigators trained through the NRSA awards are more successful in obtaining subsequent career development awards (Pion, 1996), investigators at the workshop reported finding it increasingly difficult to obtain an R01 award. The data, although partially supporting their concerns in terms of overall success rates, do not support the notion that success rates for drug abuse research differ greatly from general NIH-wide success rates. In fact, NIDA success rates, but not NIAAA, averaged higher than the overall NIH rates. Success rates for funding the R01 research project grants are declining across all NIH institutes, including NIAAA. R01 success rates for NIAAA varied between 17 percent and 32 percent between FYs 1991 and 1995, compared to 25 percent to 37 percent between FYs 1986 and 1990. At NIDA, although reduced from success rates during FY 1986–1987 (36.3 percent and 43.2 percent) and FY 1989–1990 (36.3 percent and 39.8 percent), success rates for R01 awards have stabilized around 30 percent since FY 1991 (Table 7.2).

The low number of research training and research awards made by NIDA and NIAAA is in part a result of their lower total budget for research training support (Figure 7.3); also, it is partly offset by the smaller number of applicants. Increasing research training support without increasing the availability of research project grant funding creates a frustrating discontinuity; newly trained researchers are unable to find the research support needed for career success. For example, although funding for research training at NIAAA substantially increased in 1994 and 1995, the instability of research funding in terms of R01 success rates over the past 5 years has evoked caution among promising young researchers in alcohol research (Table 7.2). The committee is concerned that further decreases in funding would prevent many scientists from going into the field or fail to sustain researchers currently employed in addiction research.

The committee found that the training budgets for NIDA and NIAAA, either as a percentage of the extramural research budget or in dollars, are low compared to other NIH institutes. NIDA's $9.3 million and NIAAA's $5.2 million training budget in FY 1995 were 2.5 percent and 2.8 percent, respectively, of their extramural research funding (Tables 7.3 and 7.4). In contrast, NHLBI spent 5 percent on training grants (the NIH average is 5 percent) and the NIMH spent 7 percent. These differences were even more pronounced before the mid-1990s, when research training funds at several of the NIH institutes were substantially increased (e.g., NIDA and NCI) from earlier levels, primarily because of mandated increases, such as support for HIV/AIDS research and research training, rather than increases in the general budget.

122

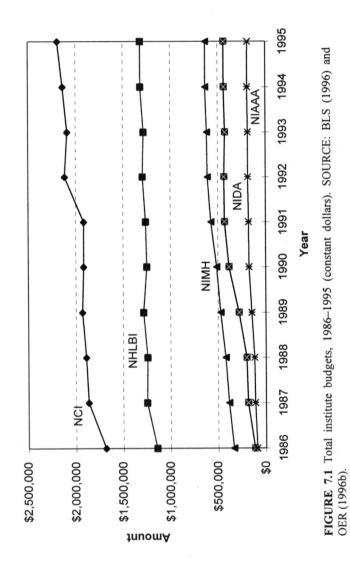

FIGURE 7.1 Total institute budgets, 1986–1995 (constant dollars). SOURCE: BLS (1996) and OER (1996b).

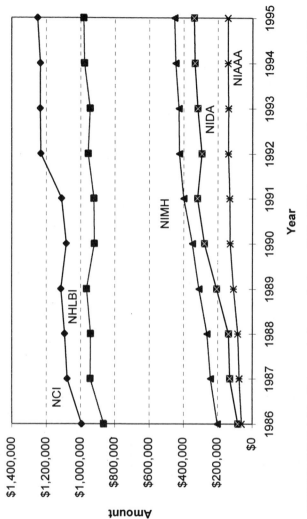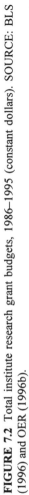

FIGURE 7.2 Total institute research grant budgets, 1986–1995 (constant dollars). SOURCE: BLS (1996) and OER (1996b).

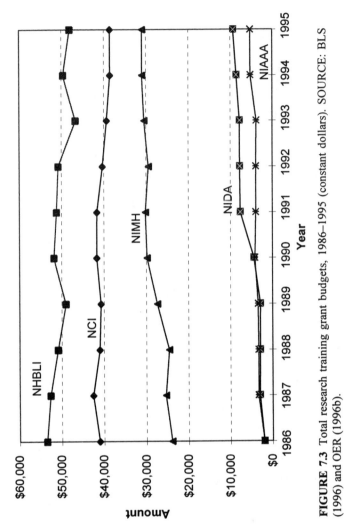

FIGURE 7.3 Total research training grant budgets, 1986–1995 (constant dollars). SOURCE: BLS (1996) and OER (1996b).

125

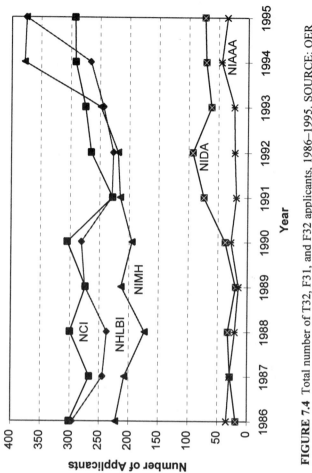

FIGURE 7.4 Total number of T32, F31, and F32 applicants, 1986–1995. SOURCE: OER (1996a).

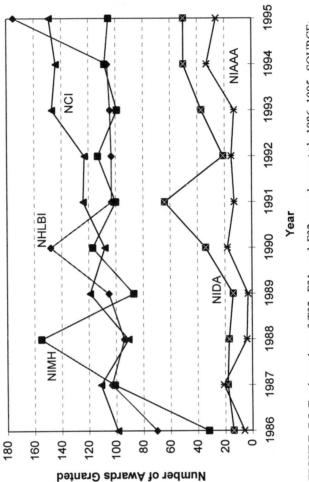

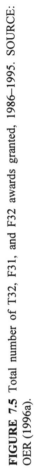

FIGURE 7.5 Total number of T32, F31, and F32 awards granted, 1986–1995. SOURCE: OER (1996a).

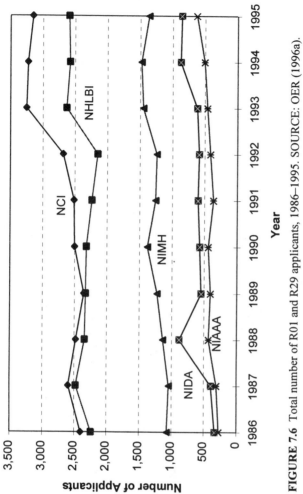

FIGURE 7.6 Total number of R01 and R29 applicants, 1986–1995. SOURCE: OER (1996a).

128

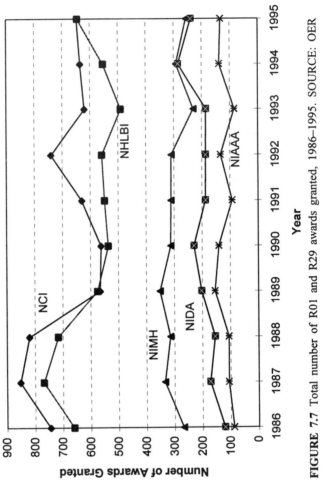

FIGURE 7.7 Total number of R01 and R29 awards granted, 1986–1995. SOURCE: OER (1996a).

TABLE 7.2 R01 Success Rates

Fiscal Year	NIH			NIAAA			NIDA		
	Applicants (Awards)	Average Size	Success Rate	Applicants (Awards)	Average Size	Success Rate	Applicants (Awards)	Average Size	Success Rate
1986	17,212 (5,408)	$135,650	31.4%	272 (88)	$116,318	32.4%	333 (121)	$142,182	36.3%
1987	15,825 (5,608)	$154,816	35.4%	282 (103)	$138,262	36.5%	387 (167)	$158,216	43.2%
1988	16,814 (5,170)	$157,707	30.7%	379 (94)	$161,564	24.8%	851 (145)	$167,614	17.0%
1989	17,257 (4,607)	$173,956	26.7%	369 (137)	$161,920	37.1%	523 (190)	$181,053	36.3%
1990	17,898 (4,112)	$186,797	23.0%	418 (134)	$215,112	32.1%	548 (218)	$211,986	39.8%
1986–1990 Total	85,006 (24,905)	$160,075	29.3%	1,720 (556)	$163,079	32.3%	2,642 (841)	$176,627	31.8%
1991	17,203 (4,709)	$198,123	27.4%	339 (85)	$239,024	25.1%	570 (172)	$236,878	30.2%
1992	17,579 (4,769)	$203,701	27.1%	394 (124)	$220,960	31.5%	551 (167)	$256,030	30.3%
1993	19,314 (4,121)	$205,394	21.3%	436 (76)	$211,342	17.4%	584 (174)	$256,580	29.8%
1994	20,573 (4,821)	$212,756	23.4%	472 (127)	$223,299	27.0%	831 (174)	$261,603	32.1%
1995	20,100 (5,001)	$228,508	24.9%	577 (119)	$239,303	20.6%	813 (267)	$274,486	27.0%
1991–1995 Total	94,769 (23,421)	$210,038	24.7%	2,218 (531)	$227,145	23.9%	3,349 (1,000)	$258,380	29.9%

SOURCE: OER (1996a).

TABLE 7.3 NIDA Research Training Funding as a Percentage of Total Extramural Research Funding (millions of dollars)

	Research Training						Percentage of Total Extramural Research
	Individual		Institutional		Total		
Year	No.	Amount	No.	Amount	No.	Amount	
1986	24	0.40	55	1.03	79	1.43	2.2
1987	36	0.67	78	1.58	114	2.25	2.0
1988	31	0.57	83	1.73	114	2.30	1.9
1989	34	0.64	80	1.73	174	2.37	1.5
1990	44	0.83	130	2.98	174	3.81	1.4
1991	73	1.26	203	5.55	276	6.81	2.1
1992	61	1.11	236	6.01	297	7.12	2.1
1993	65	1.26	237	6.11	302	7.37	2.2
1994	79	1.43	266	6.90	345	8.33	2.3
1995	63	1.67	291	7.54	374	9.31	2.5

SOURCE: IOM (1995), NIDA (1994, 1996), and OER (1996b).

TABLE 7.4 NIAAA Research Training Funding as a Percentage of Total Extramural Research Funding (millions of dollars)

	Research Training						Percentage of Total Extramural Research
	Individual		Institutional		Total		
Year	No.	Amount	No.	Amount	No.	Amount	
1986	10	0.20	61	1.23	71	1.4	2.2
1987	10	0.18	113	2.32	123	2.5	3.0
1988	10	0.19	119	2.40	129	2.6	2.8
1989	7	0.14	113	2.65	120	2.8	2.3
1990	15	0.31	132	3.27	147	3.6	2.4
1991	23	0.45	137	3.10	160	3.5	2.2
1992	18	0.37	123	3.23	141	3.6	2.1
1993	19	0.39	130	3.22	149	3.6	2.1
1994	36	0.73	147	4.31	183	5.0	2.7
1995	45	0.85	167	4.39	212	5.2	2.8

SOURCE: NIAAA (1996) and OER (1996b).

Alternatives to Federal Funding

Academic researchers rely heavily on federal funding to succeed in their careers. Another route for the young investigator pursuing a career in addiction research is through industry. The opportunity to earn higher salaries, to conduct research with large budgets, and to have ready-made collaborations attracts many young researchers who have completed their graduate or postdoctoral training. A research career in industry, however, offers a different set of career incentives and institutional environments from NIH-funded research careers in academic institutions.

Foundations provide an additional, and often innovative, pathway of support for the career development of research scientists (Box 7.2). However, there are few awards to new investigators (NRC, 1994). Foundation funding of addiction research increased from $4.4 million in 1980 to $26.4 million in 1987 (The Foundation Center, 1989), although those increases have not continued.[2] One exception is the Robert Wood Johnson Foundation (RWJF), which continues to support addiction research, primarily in the health services area. However, RWJF currently does not have any programs to recruit young investigators into addiction research. Several other foundations have supported addiction research in the past, but no longer do so, largely owing to stigma, lack of outcome measures, absence of a clear definition of their role, a belief that such funding is the responsibility of government, and changing priorities (The Foundation Center, 1989). Recently, a few foundations have begun to support young investigators in addiction research through seed money for new projects, funds to travel to conferences, or through initiatives that foster careers for young investigators. However, these programs benefit relatively few addiction researchers.

Competition with Senior Researchers

As in other fields, there is the perception in addiction research that funding favors more established researchers. A recent study of the National Research Council (NRC) (1994) found that success rates are dropping for grant ap-

---

[2]For 1993–1994, The Foundation Center's *Grants for Alcohol and Drug Abuse* lists 776 grants of $10,000 or more totaling $57,355,742 from 342 foundations. However, that figure is not comparable with the figures in The Foundation Center's 1989 report *Alcohol and Drug Abuse Funding: An Analysis of Foundation Grants, 1983–1987.* The 1993–1994 report included all grants related to alcohol and drug abuse, including prevention programs and media projects, while the 1989 report focused solely on foundation support for basic, behavioral, and clinical research of alcoholism and drug abuse. Overall, foundation support for alcohol and drug abuse research has not increased significantly in recent years (The Foundation Center, 1995, 1996).

BOX 7.2
Foundation-Funded Research: A Model Program

The "Great Neglected Diseases of Mankind" Program was established in 1978 by the Rockefeller Foundation and focused on the development of young investigators and international collaborative research. The goal of that program was to create a network of high-quality investigators who would constitute a critical mass in the field of infectious disease. The research ranged from basic through clinical investigation and field epidemiology. Support was provided for 8 years and annual meetings were held to foster communication and collaboration. The program resulted in 14 research laboratories working on the health problems of the developing world, involved 161 scientists and clinicians and 360 trainees, and resulted in publication of 1,280 articles. The total cost to the Rockefeller Foundation was $15 million. (*Lancet*, 1994; Warren and Jimenez, 1988).

---

plications submitted by younger investigators. This suggests stiffer competition with more senior researchers and lends some credence to young investigators' complaints that their research careers are constrained by "fiefdoms," where they are always in the shadow of an established senior researcher in the addiction field. However, there are no objective analyses to determine whether this field is any more, or less, driven by experienced researchers than other areas.

To meet the challenges for developing careers in addiction research, the committee recommends that:

• **The number of research career development awards should be increased, greater flexibility in duration and time-to-start of awards should be provided, and the funding priority of such awards should be advanced;**
• **The use of the B/START (Behavioral Science Track Award for Rapid Transition) mechanism now at NIMH and NIDA to provide seed money for young investigators should be expanded;**
• **Programs for student-directed summer research should be established by NIDA and NIAAA;**
• **Industry and private foundations should cooperate with universities to provide supplemental funds for career development and research support of young investigators, especially during transition periods between awards, or to provide partial salary support for clinical researchers;**
• **Increases should be made in the percentage of NIDA and NIAAA extramural research funding spent on training programs to reach the NIH institute average (currently 5 percent to 6 percent), funds for which should *not* be redirected from the research budgets of these institutes;**
• **Jointly sponsored programs (e.g., government, industry, private foundations, academia) to support research training should be established**

with clear roles and responsibilities for the participation of each institution; and

• NIDA and NIAAA should explore the possibility of providing bridging support for promising young investigators to assist in the transition from K01 and R29 to R01 funding.

Special Problems for Clinical Investigators

The problem of attracting M.D.s, M.D./Ph.D.s, and Ph.D.s into a research career has been noted in other studies (IOM, 1994; IOM, 1995; NRC, 1994; Pincus et al., 1995). In drug addiction research, attracting clinical researchers and sustaining their careers is even more difficult (IOM, 1995). Although both NIDA and NIAAA have implemented efforts to use the K20 awards to attract more M.D.s and M.D./Ph.D.s into the field, very few have been awarded. NIDA increased the number of M.D./Ph.D. clinical research awards from 3 in FY 1990 to 10 in FY 1995, while NIAAA has continued to fund only 1 or 2 M.D./Ph.D. clinical researchers a year.

Level of Stipends

As with all federally funded pre- and postdoctoral training awards, the level of the stipends poses another type of barrier for young investigators. Recent increases in stipends for NIH predoctoral researchers and junior postdoctoral researchers have brought such awards more in line with other federal and non-federal programs; stipends rose from $8,800 to $10,008 per year for predoctoral researchers, and from $19,700 to $20,700 for those with at least 1 full year of postdoctoral experience (NIH, 1992, 1996b). Despite these increases, these stipends are extremely low compared to salaries for individuals of comparable ages in other careers.

The low funding level of awards is often a particular barrier for attracting physicians who want to be clinical investigators. The maximum salary for a fourth- or fifth-year postgraduate M.D. investigator in basic research is about $30,000, while an M.D. taking a junior faculty position may earn between $70,000 to $80,000 (AAMC, 1995). Basic health insurance and other benefits are also very limited. Under the current system, payback of education-related debt must begin in the third year of postgraduate training, and most graduate and postgraduates have significant debt (AAMC, 1995).[3] To alleviate the debt burden, research training is sometimes eliminated to allow earlier entry into practice, and many M.D. investigators moonlight to supplement the low salaries

---

[3]The mean personal debt for graduating and postgraduate medical students in 1995 was $85,000 (AAMC, 1995).

of research positions (NRC, 1994). This is also a problem for Ph.D.-trained clinical researchers (IOM, 1994). These financial pressures may detract from their enthusiasm for a research career.

Competing Demands

Another barrier for many clinical researchers is trying to balance teaching, clinical, and research responsibilities. Academic departments have exerted added pressure for many investigators to increase their clinical efforts, impairing their ability to pursue research. Combined with shifts in health care funding and in support by the federal and state governments, excessively heavy clinical workloads are likely to have significant consequences for future research careers. As one young M.D./Ph.D. investigator stated, "There is always tension between the need to deliver services for my department while at the same time trying to keep my research going." Another commented on "the challenge of protecting the time for research through grant dollars that is becoming increasingly difficult due to grant funding limitations." The demands of clinical practice place enormous pressure on the clinical researcher's schedule.

To encourage excellence in clinical research on the problems of addiction, the committee recommends that:

• **The federal government should establish a debt deferral or forgiveness program for scientists conducting clinical research in drug addiction or treating persons with drug abuse in publicly funded settings; and**
• **Federal funds should be made available from NIH, SAMSHA, HRSA, or AHCPR to provide training for primary care physicians (e.g., obstetricians, family physicians, and internists) to recognize, treat effectively, or refer patients with drug abuse problems.**

Integration and Collaboration

In recent years, there has been increasing recognition that the behavioral sciences and neurosciences have advanced the field of addiction research and treatment (IOM, 1996). The behavioral sciences have contributed to our understanding of the complex behaviors of initiation, maintenance, cessation, and relapse to addiction, while the neurosciences have described neural mechanisms and common reward pathways responsible for addictive behaviors. That research may illuminate the underlying causes of addiction and provide theory-guided direction for the development of treatment and prevention strategies. Integration and collaboration of these research perspectives will benefit all types of research, basic and applied.

Unfortunately, integrative and collaborative research tends to be the exception rather than the standard. For example, agencies tend to be oriented toward funding research programs that are drug-or issue-specific. Requests for proposals (RFPs) and grants reflect the interests of the funding agency and are often focused on a specific problem and/or are discipline-specific. Study sections tend to be comprised of individuals knowledgeable about one discipline or field of research, and awards are granted to studies that are based on criteria that do not include or give priority to interdisciplinary research. In addition, the organization of most universities into disciplinary departments makes interdisciplinary research difficult to conduct and manage (NAS, 1995). Collaborative efforts within institutes or agencies are often impeded by proprietary concerns, conceptual differences, funding conflicts, and competition. Although those traditional mechanisms are important for funding research in any area, it would appear that in some instances a break with tradition is necessary to deal with interdisciplinary and collaborative research.

Effective and productive multidisciplinary collaboration is difficult to achieve, but is possible when there is a commitment by scientists and clinicians in the field to support collaborative efforts involving basic, clinical, and behavioral science. In light of the recent advances in the field and the importance of collaborative and integrative research efforts to address the problems of addiction and relapse, the committee recommends that:

- **Funding institutions, such as the government and private foundations, should develop program funding mechanisms (e.g., Requests for Applications [RFAs], annual conferences, symposia) to foster collaborative exchanges of information and research, such as the scientific breakthroughs that occur during drug development;**
- **Universities with faculty engaged in addiction research should undertake a comprehensive review of the support and resources available for collaborative efforts within and outside the university, particularly those collaborative efforts which involve multiple disciplines; administrators should develop a plan to share resources and facilities both within and across institutions and specify criteria for access;**
- **Funding agencies, such as the government and private foundations, should focus on new integrative opportunities (e.g., drug addiction etiology and medications) through using the combined strengths of participating institutions, including government, industry, private foundations, multidisciplinary centers, and Academic Centers of Excellence;**
- **NIH should review the composition of Initial Review Groups (IRGs) to ensure that there is appropriate representation across necessary disciplines;**

- **NIDA and NIAAA should consider establishing additional mechanisms or expanding R03 awards for individual investigator awards that support innovative, high-risk, interdisciplinary research; and**
- **Additional sources of resources to increase and support integrative and collaborative efforts in addiction research should be considered by Congress; for example, the percentage of the budget of the White House Office of National Drug Control Policy earmarked for research should be increased substantially as part of coordinated strategy to make drug abuse and addiction research a national priority.**

REFERENCES

AAMC (Association of American Medical Colleges). 1995. *Minority Students in Medical Education: Facts and Figures IX.* Washington, DC: Association of American Medical Colleges.

BLS (Bureau of Labor Statistics). 1996. *Consumer Price Index: All Urban Consumers, U.S. City Average, All Items—1913–1995.* Washington, DC: Bureau of Labor Statistics.

The Foundation Center. 1989. *Alcohol and Drug Abuse Funding: An Analysis of Foundation Grants 1983–1987.* New York: The Foundation Center.

The Foundation Center. 1995. *Grants for Alcohol and Drug Abuse, 1995–1996.* New York: The Foundation Center.

The Foundation Center. 1996. Personal communication with S Qureshi. The Foundation Center. July 8.

IOM (Institute of Medicine). 1994. *Careers in Clinical Research: Obstacles and Opportunities.* Washington, DC: National Academy Press.

IOM. 1995. *The Development of Medications for the Treatment of Opiate and Cocaine Addictions.* Washington, DC: National Academy Press.

IOM. 1996. *Pathways of Addiction: Opportunities in Drug Abuse Research.* Washington, DC: National Academy Press.

Lancet. 1994. Proposal quality or product quality? *Lancet* 344:488–489.

Mervis J. 1996. NSF to take closer look at how support shapes careers. *Science* 272:806.

NAS (National Academy of Sciences). 1995. *Allocating Federal Funds for Science and Technology.* Washington, DC: National Academy Press.

NHLBI (National Heart, Lung, and Blood Institute). 1994. *Morbidity and Mortality: Chartbook on Cardiovascular, Lung, and Blood Diseases.* Washington, DC: National Heart, Lung, and Blood Institute.

NIAAA (National Institute on Alcoholism and Alcohol Abuse). 1996. *National Institute on Alcohol Abuse and Alcoholism Funding History, 1986–1995.* Rockville, MD: National Institute on Alcohol Abuse and Alcoholism.

NIDA (National Institute on Drug Abuse). 1994. *National Institute on Drug Abuse 1995 Budget Estimate.* Rockville, MD: National Institute on Drug Abuse.

NIDA. 1996. *NIDA Research Training History, 1986–1995.* Rockville, MD: National Institute on Drug Abuse.

NIH (National Institutes of Health). 1992. National research service award—Institutional grants. Request for Applications (RFA) HS-93-02. *NIH Guide* 21(38):October 23.

NIH. 1996a. Personal communication with Kimberly Garr. Office of Financial Management. June 4.

NIH. 1996b. NIH national research service awards for individual postdoctoral fellows guidelines. *NIH Guide* 25(31):September 20.

NIH. 1996c. *National Institutes of Health: Grants and Contracts.* [http://www.nih.gov/grants]. September.

NIH. 1997. Personal communication with Robert Feaga. Office of Financial Management. May 27.

NRC (National Research Council). 1994. *The Funding of Young Investigators in the Biological and Biomedical Sciences.* Washington, DC: National Academy Press.

OER (Office of Extramural Research, National Institutes of Health). 1996a. *NIH Competing Research Project Applications: Number of Applicants and Awardees for Each Award by Year and Institute, 1970–1995.* Prepared for the Committee to Identify Strategies to Raise the Profile of Substance Abuse and Alcoholism Research. Rockville, MD: Division of Computer Research and Technology, Office of Extramural Research, National Institutes of Health. May.

OER. 1996b. *Institute and Center Research Training Budgets as a Percentage of Their Budgets for NIH Extramural Research and Development Grants, FY 1995.* Rockville, MD: Office of Extramural Research, National Institutes of Health.

Pincus HA, Haviland MG, Dial TH, Hendryx MS. 1995. The relationship of postdoctoral research training to current research activities of faculty in academic departments of psychiatry. *The American Journal of Psychiatry* 152(4):596–601.

Pion G. 1996. *Analysis of Characteristics and Outcomes for NRSA Trainees and Fellows Supported by NIAAA and NIDA.* Nashville, TN: Vanderbilt University and Office of Research Training, National Institutes of Health.

Rice DP. 1995. Personal communication to the Institute of Medicine. University of California at San Francisco. February.

Varmus H. 1995. *Disease-Specific Estimates of Direct and Indirect Costs of Illness and NIH Support.* Bethesda, MD: Office of the Director, National Institutes of Health.

Warren KS, Jimenez C. 1988. *The Great Neglected Diseases of Mankind Biomedical Research Network.* New York: The Rockefeller Foundation.

8

Public Perceptions, Public Policies

This short chapter summarizes some of the key discussions concerning how drug abuse is viewed in the society and the implications of those views. These discussions occurred throughout the committee's deliberations, but received special attention at the committee's March 1996 workshop (Appendix A; see also Appendix I).

Although there have been many scientific advances in knowledge of drug addiction, the public's perceptions and understanding lag far behind (see time line in Appendix E). If the goal is to increase interest in and support for careers in addiction research, it is essential to communicate current scientific knowledge effectively to the public at large. Educating the public begins in schools and is carried further through the media and other mechanisms.

STIGMA

Even after years of public statements that drug addiction is a disease, many continue to subscribe to a moralistic view of addiction (Miller, 1991) and to see addicted people as immoral, weak-willed, or as having a character defect requiring punishment or incarceration. This stigma may serve a useful function to the extent that it may discourage some individuals from starting to use these drugs. However, stigmatizing any disease keeps some afflicted individuals from getting help for themselves and often prevents family, friends, and employers from knowledging the existence of a problem and urging a loved one or colleague to seek treatment.

The stereotype that drug abusers could change their behavior if they were sufficiently motivated is inconsistent with understanding the complex multiple factors involved in addiction. When policymakers view drug abusers as untreatable or undeserving of public support, treatment programs, insurance coverage, and research and training programs may be underfunded or abolished.

Undervalued Area of Research

The stigma associated with drug addiction has directly deterred young investigators who might otherwise be interested in pursuing careers in addiction research and treatment. Their frustration was expressed forcefully and consistently at the March 1996 workshop. For example, one of the new investigators in attendance said, "The biggest problem specific to drug abuse is one of public perceptions. Many times in my career, I have been asked by people outside science, 'Why are you studying drug abuse? Why don't you study something important like cancer?' "

In addition to the discouraging words of friends, families, and colleagues, addiction researchers described concrete reminders of the low status of their field. One new investigator described the "rusting trailer" where their research offices were located; another described how addicted patients were relegated to outbuildings because they were considered undesirable and not wanted in the main medical facility.

As a result of stigma, the realities of studying often difficult and sometimes frightening patients, and the lack of public funding and support, addiction research is often an undervalued area of inquiry with low visibility, and many scientists and clinicians choose other disciplines in which to develop their careers (IOM, 1995). In addition, many believe the field suffers from a lack of prestige stemming from what is seen as a lower quality of some of the research. These perceptions stem from several factors, including a lack of understanding about the complexities arising from multiple determinants of addiction, the difficulties involved in conducting clinical and behavioral research in this field, and other research issues, such as the regulation of drugs and confidentiality requirements (IOM, 1995, 1996). Investigators in drug abuse research are often paid less than their peers in other fields (IOM, 1995).

ADVOCACY

In considering the importance of advocacy groups to growth of other fields, the role of anti-tobacco groups, treatment providers' groups, and others that advocate better drug and alcohol abuse prevention and treatment should not be underestimated. Yet, unlike other fields in which patient groups provide a strong voice for research, there is very little heard from people who suffer from addictive disorders, particularly if illicit drugs are involved, and a certain hesitancy on the part of families to speak out because of stigma.

The National Alliance of Methadone Advocates (NAMA) is one advocacy organization that encompasses methadone maintenance patients, health care professionals, and other supporters of high-quality methadone maintenance treatment. NAMA's goals are to eliminate discrimination against methadone patients, create a more positive image about methadone maintenance treatment, help preserve patients' dignity and their rights, make treatment available on demand to every person who needs it, and empower methadone patients with a strong public voice (NAMA, 1996). NAMA is one organization composed of individuals with addiction problems and their supporters that provides a working example of how those most affected by addiction can become advocates for themselves.

The willingness to expose oneself to public scrutiny is a critical part of the formation of strong advocacy groups. The willingness to "go public" and organize is severely inhibited by the stigma resulting from the behavior changes induced by intoxicating drugs, the assumption of willful self-destruction associated with drug abuse, and the public perception of addicts as disreputable and hopeless. Further, for those addicted to drugs that are illegal, there are both real and perceived dangers in becoming involved in an advocacy organization that could bring one to the attention of law enforcement officials.

Celebrities often provide important visibility and access for an advocacy agenda, such as AIDS and spinal cord injuries. Although some high-profile persons, including Betty Ford and Carroll O'Connor, have spoken out about addiction and worked to increase public understanding, openness from a variety of celebrities about these problems and how they affect individuals and families will be a continuing need and potent force for changing public attitudes.

Many disease-oriented advocacy groups are able to mobilize behind the hope for a vaccine or a cure, even though research tends to produce only small, incremental improvements in the management of a chronic disease. Because many people see addiction as a defect of will, it is often difficult for advocates to rally behind a "race for the cure" or vaccine.

One difficult problem is that other advocacy groups with similar interests have refused to align themselves with the field of drug addiction. For example, the dual diagnosis of drug dependence and depression is quite common, but advocacy groups for depression are reluctant to form coalitions with advocates supporting treatment and research for persons with addictive diseases. Instead, these groups often end up competing for research and treatment dollars.

A MODEL FOR UNDERSTANDING
THE EDUCATIONAL AND PUBLIC BARRIERS

The committee examined the relationships among the barriers to determine their effect on the field of addiction research. A model showing the relationships among the individual barriers is depicted in Figure 8.1. The figure illustrates, for example, the connection between negative perceptions and advocacy efforts; it shows that stigma can ultimately influence research integration and collaboration. Finally, the figure identifies the barriers and their relationships, which in turn provides a basis for articulating the strategies necessary to overcome those barriers.

STRATEGIES

Inadequacies in education about addictive drugs and addiction and the pervasive stigma attached to those involved in careers in addiction research as well as those who have problems of abuse and addiction pose serious barriers for careers in addiction research and treatment. The lack of opportunities for integrative and collaborative research, the inadequacy of training and education opportunities, and limited funding levels are also significant barriers. The committee has identified these barriers and strategies to overcome them based on members' own judgment, information gleaned from the workshop, and additional information acquired in the course of this study.

Informing the Public

New approaches should be adopted to help the public in general and educators and policymakers in particular to better understand the neurobiological and behavioral basis of addiction and the effectiveness of treatment. These approaches should focus on providing a basic vocabulary and a basic level of understanding about brain reward circuitry and the behavioral systems that are relevant to the actions of addictive drugs and treatment strategies.

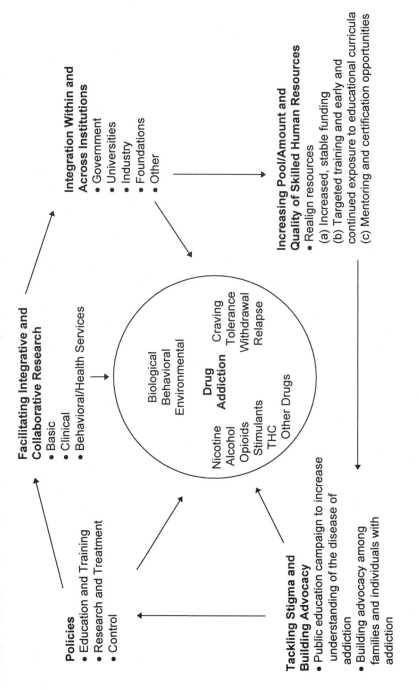

FIGURE 8.1 Critical links in the strategies for raising the profile of addiction research.

Toward this end, the committee recommends that:

- **Public education campaigns should be based on an interdisciplinary view of addiction and emphasize treatment effectiveness, as well as include descriptions of the role of brain physiology and function (e.g., pain systems, anxiety circuits, mood systems, and behavioral and psychosocial aspects).**

A goal of the campaign could be to redefine drug addiction as a preventable and treatable brain disease influenced by a complex set of behaviors that may be the result of genetic, biological, psychosocial, and environmental interactions, and to emphasize the ways drugs can fundamentally alter neural or brain function. A key to increased understanding of the kinds of changes associated with repeated drug use may be the concept that these drugs can capture control of brain mechanisms that control motivations and emotions (i.e., basic drives, such as anger, fear, anxiety, pain, and depression). Information should focus on the idea that drugs can interact with systems regulating these basic drive states through effects on receptors in the brain and neural circuitry (Chapter 3).

Although the public's views cannot be changed overnight, educational efforts should provide the public with the basis for appreciating that drugs which act on basic brain mechanisms are not inherently "good" or "bad" but can lead to fundamental alterations in neural or brain function when used inappropriately. In addition, information should be provided to help the public understand that inappropriate drug use can deregulate or disrupt the normal functions of brain systems. This deregulation can be long-lasting; even well after drug use stops, various environmental and emotional triggers can bring about powerful urges to reintroduce drug use (i.e., craving).

In addition, school- or community-based health education programs should be encouraged to address the issues of drug addiction (described above). They should be addressed at appropriate age levels in schools, particularly those with health education and prevention programs.

A campaign for addiction education should include Ad Council initiatives, private and public funding of efforts to develop educational programs for schools or community-based and adult education programs, educational computer programs, and public television and other media communications. In particular, science writers should be educated through press conferences and public symposia.

The Role of Advocacy Groups

Advocacy groups have been particularly effective in generating support for health research and in helping to set research agendas. For example, the stigma associated with alcoholism has seriously decreased over the past 50 years in large part as a result of the strong voices and openness of people suffering from alcoholism and their families. The committee believes it is essential to engage more recovered people and their families in the strengthening and formation of organizations that could form a national advocacy network for addiction research.

The families of nicotine, alcohol, and illegal drug users could expand their efforts to build stronger advocacy groups to help destigmatize addictive disease. It may prove wise to begin with families of individuals addicted to legal drugs, because these are more acceptable to the public, and then enlist individuals whose relatives abuse illegal drugs. In advocacy, it is important to emphasize what works and why and to link research and treatment to other areas, such as mental health. And to be effective, messages need to be consistent in definitions and vocabulary and presented in lay terms.

Advocacy can be assisted by private foundations, industry, universities, and other professional organizations as well as physicians and scientists in leadership roles. They can translate research findings and new clinical developments for existing advocacy groups and community leaders, and emphasize the importance of a strong research infrastructure.

Specific strategies to increase public understanding and reduce stigma should include:

• Increasing communications with the media to report accurate, reliable, and timely information about research findings to the widest spectrum of government and industry officials and to the broader public;

• Disseminating scientific information to increase the public's awareness of the neurobiological and behavioral underpinnings of addictive disease, the value of treatment, and the importance of research;

• Forging an alliance between local citizens' groups and scientists to conduct local symposia at which the public can hear presentations by scientists;

• Strengthening existing grassroots organizations and organizing new groups;

• Seeking funding for science writers;

• Aggressively seeking increased support for research on nicotine, alcohol, and illegal drugs;

• Increasing the focus on addiction research within existing organizations that advocate on behalf of addiction treatment and services; and

- Identifying and seeking involvement by high-profile individuals affected by addiction to discuss the scientific basis of the treatment of addictive disorders and the need for new research.

To address these challenges, the committee recommends:

- **Consumer and other advocacy groups should be encouraged to strengthen their focus on the need for research on the causes, prevention, and treatment of addictive disorders.**
- **Liaison relationships and joint activities should be explored among advocacy groups to increase public understanding of addictive disorders. Activities could include meetings of representatives of provider groups, state and local health departments, and established grassroots advocacy groups, to develop cohesive, workable strategies to accomplish change.**

REFERENCES

IOM (Institute of Medicine). 1995. *The Development of Medications for the Treatment of Opiate and Cocaine Addictions*. Washington, DC: National Academy Press.

IOM. 1996. *Pathways of Addiction: Opportunities in Drug Abuse Research*. Washington, DC: National Academy Press.

Miller NS. 1991. Drug and alcohol addiction as a disease. In: Miller NS, ed. *Comprehensive Handbook of Drug and Alcohol Addiction*. New York: Marcel Dekker, Inc. Pp. 295–309.

NAMA (National Alliance of Methadone Advocates). 1996. *Factsheet* [http://www.nama.org]. October.

Appendixes

A

Workshop Agenda

INSTITUTE OF MEDICINE
NATIONAL ACADEMY OF SCIENCES

Committee to Identify Strategies to Raise the Profile of Substance Abuse and Alcoholism Research
Workshop on Raising the Profile of Substance Abuse and Alcoholism Research

March 28–29, 1996
Lecture Room, National Academy of Sciences
2101 Constitution Avenue, N.W.
Washington, D.C.

WORKSHOP AGENDA
Day One—March 28, 1996

8:15–8:30 a.m.	*Opening Remarks* Dr. Stanley Watson, Committee Vice Chair
8:30–11:00	*Panel Sessions*
8:30–8:50	**Panel One: Young Investigators (Basic Research)** Facilitator: Dr. Richard Tsien
8:50–9:15	**Discussion**
9:15–9:35	**Panel Two: Young Investigators (Clinical Research)** Facilitator: Dr. Ting Kai Li
9:35–10:00	**Discussion**

10:00–10:10	**Break**
10:10–10:35	**Panel Three: Young Investigators (Health Services, Community, Behavioral Research)** Facilitator: Dr. Sally Satel
10:35–11:00	**Discussion**
11:00–12:40	***Plenary Session:***
11:00–11:30	**Dr. Avram Goldstein, Professor Emeritus of Pharmacology, Stanford University**
11:30–11:50	**Questions, Answers, and Discussion**
11:50–12:20	**Dr. Ivan Diamond, Professor and Vice Chair, Department of Neurology, University of California at San Francisco**
12:20–12:40	**Questions, Answers, and Discussion**
12:40–1:30	**Lunch**
1:30–3:30	***Working Groups Meeting*** Neurosciences/Animal Models Cofacilitators: Drs. Marc Caron and Judith Walters Human Subjects Research Cofacilitators: Drs. Sharon Hall and William Schmidt
3:30–3:45	**Break**
3:45–5:00	***Reports and Discussion of Breakout Groups***
5:00–5:30	***Closing Synopsis and Workshop Summary—Day I***
5:30–6:30	***Reception***

Day Two—March 29, 1996

8:30–8:45 a.m.	*Welcome and Purpose of Second Day* Dr. Stanley Watson, Committee Vice Chair
8:45–12:00	*Lessons Learned*
8:45–9:15	**Depression** Herbert Pardes, M.D., Vice President for Health Sciences and Dean of the Faculty of Medicine, Columbia University
9:15–9:20	**Brief Question-and-Answer Period**
9:20–9:50	**Epilepsy** Dominick Purpura, M.D., Dean, Albert Einstein College of Medicine
9:50–9:55	**Brief Question-and-Answer Period**
9:55–10:25	**Breast Cancer** Kay Dickersin, Ph.D., Assistant Professor, University of Maryland
10:25–10:30	**Brief Question-and-Answer Period**
10:30–10:45	**Break**
10:45–12:00	***Discussion of Lessons Learned and Other Innovative Strategies for Raising the Profile of Substance Abuse and Alcoholism Research***
12:00	***Workshop Adjourned***

B

Workshop Contributors and Participants

INSTITUTE OF MEDICINE
NATIONAL ACADEMY OF SCIENCES

Committee to Identify Strategies to Raise the Profile of Substance Abuse and Alcoholism Research
Workshop on Raising the Profile of Substance Abuse and Alcoholism Research

March 28–29, 1996
Lecture Room, National Academy of Sciences
2101 Constitution Avenue, N.W.
Washington, D.C.

Jill U. Adams, Ph.D.
Research Assistant Professor
Department of Psychiatry
New York University

Gina Agostinelli, Ph.D.
Postdoctoral Fellow
Prevention Research Center
Berkeley, CA

Bruce Alberts, Ph.D.
President
National Academy of Sciences
Washington, D.C.

Amelia M. Arria, Ph.D.
Assistant Public Health Scientist
Johns Hopkins University

Brad Austin
Center for Substance Abuse
Treatment
Substance Abuse and Mental
Health Services Administration
Rockville, MD

Thomas Babor, Ph.D., M.P.H.
Scientific Director
Alcohol Research Center
Farmington, CT

James Baxendale, Ph.D.
Deputy Director
Quality Assurance and Case
Management Programs
National Association of State
Alcohol and Drug Abuse
Directors, Inc.
Washington, D.C.

153

Michael J. Bohn, M.D.
Assistant Professor of Psychiatry
University of Wisconsin
  Medical School

Joseph V. Brady, Ph.D.
Professor of Behavioral Biology
  and Professor of Neuroscience
Behavioral Biology Research
  Center
Johns Hopkins University School
  of Medicine

Jeanine Bussiere, Ph.D., DABT
Scientist
Genentech, Inc.
San Francisco, CA

Joseph Califano, M.D.
Center on Addiction and Substance
  Abuse
New York, NY

Anne Carney, Ph.D.
Associate Professor
Alcohol Research Center
University of Connecticut Health
  Center
Farmington, CT

Richard Chipkin, Ph.D.
Research Scientist
Schering-Plough Research
Kenilworth, NJ

Jean Comolli
Science Policy Branch
National Institute on Drug Abuse
Rockville, MD

Timothy Condon, Ph.D.
Chief, Science Policy Branch
National Institute on Drug Abuse
Rockville, MD

Rena Convissor
Center for the Advancement of
  Health
Washington, D.C.

Shawn Cooper, Ph.D.
Clinical Research Division in
  Substance Abuse
Wayne State University
Detroit, MI

Joseph Coyle, M.D.
Professor of Neurosciences
Harvard Medical School

Roger Detels, M.D.
Director, NIDA Training Center
University of California at Los
  Angeles

Ivan Diamond, M.D., Ph.D.
Professor and Vice Chair
Department of Neurology
University of California at San
  Francisco

Kay Dickersin, Ph.D.
Assistant Professor
Department of Epidemiology
  and Preventive Medicine
University of Maryland School
  of Medicine

Karen Downey, Ph.D.
Clinical Research Division in
  Substance Abuse
Wayne State University
Detroit, MI

Ronith Elk, Ph.D.
Assistant Professor
University of Texas at Houston
Health Sciences Center

Mark Feinberg, M.D., Ph.D.
Medical Officer, Office of AIDS
 Research
Bethesda, MD

Robert Freedman, M.D.
Professor and Director
Center for Neurosciences and
 Schizophrenia
University of Colorado Health
 Sciences Center

Richard K. Fuller, M.D.
Director, Division of Clinical and
 Prevention Research
National Institute on Alcohol
 Abuse and Alcoholism
Rockville, MD

Marc Galanter, M.D.
Professor of Psychiatry
Director, Division of Alcoholism
 and Drug Abuse
New York University Medical
 Center

Julie Gilbert
Medical Student
Harvard University

Avram Goldstein, M.D.
Professor Emeritus of
 Pharmacology
Department of Molecular Biology
Stanford University

Enoch Gordis, M.D.
Director
National Institute on Alcohol
 Abuse and Alcoholism
Rockville, MD

Mark Greenwald, Ph.D.
Clinical Research Division in
 Substance Abuse
Wayne State University
Detroit, MI

Neil E. Grunberg, Ph.D.
Department of Medical and
 Clinical Psychology
Uniformed Services University of
 the Health Sciences
Bethesda, MD

R. Adron Harris, Ph.D.
Professor of Pharmacology
University of Colorado Health
 Sciences Center

Henrick J. Harwood
Senior Manager
Lewin-VHI, Inc.
Fairfax, VA

Ken Hoffman, M.D., M.P.H.
Director, Center for Addiction
 Medicine
Uniformed Services University of
 the Health Sciences
Bethesda, MD

John Hopper, M.D.
Clinical Research Division in
 Substance Abuse
Wayne State University
Detroit, MI

Sari Izenwasser, Ph.D.
Psychobiology Section
Addiction Research Center
National Institute on Drug Abuse
Baltimore, MD

Paul S. Jellinek
Vice President
The Robert Wood Johnson
Foundation
Princeton, NJ

Chris-Ellyn Johanson, Ph.D.
Clinical Research Division in
Substance Abuse
Wayne State University
Detroit, MI

Sara Jones, Ph.D.
Department of Cell Biology
Duke University Medical Center

Rhonda Jones-Webb, Dr.P.H.
Assistant Professor
University of Minnesota School
of Public Health

Linda Kaplan
Executive Director
National Association of
Alcoholism and Drug Abuse
Counselors
Arlington, VA

Henry Khachaturian
Associate Director, Division of
Neuroscience and Behavioral
Science
National Institute of Mental Health
Rockville, MD

Nancy Kilpatrick
Public Health Analyst
Center for Substance Abuse
Treatment
Rockville, MD

George R. King, Ph.D.
Assistant Research Professor
Duke University Medical Center

Deborah Kreiss, Ph.D.
Neurophysiological Pharmacology
Section
National Institute of Neurological
Disorders and Stroke
Rockville, MD

Jill Kuennen, M.A.
Clinical Research Division in
Substance Abuse
Wayne State University
Detroit, MI

David Kupfer, M.D.
Professor and Chairman of
Psychiatry
University of Pittsburgh School of
Medicine

Alan I. Leshner, Ph.D.
Director
National Institute on Drug Abuse
Rockville, MD

Jay Levy, M.D.
Cancer Research Institute
University of California at San
Francisco

David Lewis, M.D.
Center for Alcohol and Addiction
Studies
Brown University

Ed Linehan
Program Analyst
National Institute on Alcohol
  Abuse and Alcoholism
Rockville, MD

Stephen W. Long
Director, Office of Policy Analysis
National Institute on Alcohol
  Abuse and Alcoholism
Rockville, MD

Juan Lopez, M.D.
Mental Health Research Institute
University of Michigan

Alan Marlatt, Ph.D.
Professor of Psychology and
  Director
Addictive Behavior Research
  Center
University of Washington

James McKay, Ph.D.
Assistant Professor
Treatment Research Center
University of Pennsylvania

A. Thomas McLellan, Ph.D.
Treatment Research Institute, Inc.
University of Pennsylvania

Robert F. Moore
Division of Research Grants
National Institutes of Health
Bethesda, MD

Roland Moore, Ph.D.
Research Anthropologist
Prevention Research Center
Berkeley, CA

Geoffrey Mumford, Ph.D.
Department of Psychiatry
Johns Hopkins Bay View Campus

Helen Munoz
Special Assistant to the
  Administrator
Substance Abuse and Mental
  Health Services Administration
Rockville, MD

Peggy Murray, M.S.W.
Coordinator, Research and
  Training
National Institute on Alcohol
  Abuse and Alcoholism
Rockville, MD

Peter Nathan, Ph.D.
Department of Psychology
University of Iowa

Douglas Novins, M.D.
National Center on Alcohol
University of Colorado

Christine M. Ohannessian, Ph.D.
Assistant Professor
Department of Kinesiology and
  Health Education
University of Texas at Austin

Herbert Pardes, M.D.
Vice President for Health Sciences
  and Dean of the Faculty of
  Medicine
Columbia University

Elizabeth Parks
Doctoral Candidate
Columbia University
Society for Seamen's Children
New York, NY

Carol Paronis, Ph.D.
New England Regional Primate
  Research Center
Division on Behavioral Biology
Harvard Medical School
Southborough, MA

Robert Phillips
National Association of
  Alcoholism and Drug Abuse
  Counselors
Roswell, NM

Nancy Piotrowski, Ph.D.
Alcohol Research Group
University of California at
  Berkeley

Dominick P. Purpura, M.D.
Dean
Albert Einstein College of
  Medicine
New York, NY

Malcolm S. Reid, Ph.D.
Department of Psychiatry
University of California at San
  Francisco

Rudy Richardson, Sc.D.
Professor and Director
Toxicology Program
University of Michigan

John L.R. Rubenstein, M.D., Ph.D.
Associate Professor
Department of Psychiatry
University of California at San
  Francisco

Stanley Sacks, Ph.D.
Deputy Director
Institute for Special Population
  Research
National Development and
  Research Institutes, Inc.
New York, NY

Christine A. Sannerud, Ph.D.
Drug Sciences Specialist
Office of Diversion Control
Drug and Chemical Evaluation
  Section
Drug Enforcement Administration
Washington, D.C.

Walter T. Schaffer, Ph.D.
NIH Research Training Officer
Bethesda, MD

Eugene Schoener, Ph.D.
Clinical Research Division in
  Substance Abuse
Wayne State University
Detroit, MI

Kory Schuh, Ph.D.
Clinical Research Division in
  Substance Abuse
Wayne State University
Detroit, MI

Leslie Schuh, Ph.D.
Clinical Research Division in
  Substance Abuse
Wayne State University
Detroit, MI

Terry K. Schultz, M.D.
American Society of Addiction
  Medicine
Arlington, VA

Charles R. Schuster, Ph.D.
Director, Clinical Research
Division on Substance Abuse
Wayne State University
Detroit, MI

Edward M. Sellers, M.D., Ph.D.
Addiction Research Foundation
Toronto, Ontario
Canada

Kenneth I. Shine, M.D.
President
Institute of Medicine
Washington, D.C.

Lisa V. Smith, M.P.H.
Department of Epidemiology
University of California at Los
  Angeles
School of Public Health

Penni St. Hilaire
Senior Program Management
  Officer
Center for Substance Abuse
  Treatment
Rockville, MD

Robert B. Stewart, Ph.D.
Department of Psychology
Indiana University

Carla Storr
Doctoral Candidate
Johns Hopkins University

Boris Tabakoff, Ph.D.
Professor and Chairman
Department of Pharmacology
University of Colorado School of
  Medicine

Thomas Tatham, Ph.D.
Department of Behavioral
  Pharmacology
Uniformed Services University of
  the Health Sciences
Bethesda, MD

Paul J. Tiseo, Ph.D.
Assistant Director
Clinical Research
Eisai America, Inc.
Teaneck, NJ

Alison Trinkoff, D.Sc.
Associate Professor
Univerisity of Maryland School
  of Nursing

Keith A. Trujillo, Ph.D.
Psychology Program
California State University at San
  Marcos

Jaylan Turkkan, Ph.D.
Chief, Behavioral Sciences Branch
National Institute on Drug Abuse
Rockville, MD

C. Fernando Valenzuela, M.D.,
  Ph.D.
Postdoctoral Fellow
University of Colorado Health
  Sciences Center

Stuart R. Varon
Medical Director
Johns Hopkins Children's Mental
  Health Center

Delia M. Vasquez, M.D.
Mental Health Research Institute
University of Michigan

Sophia Vinogradov, M.D.
Assistant Professor
Department of Psychiatry
University of California at San
  Francisco

David Warren
North Carolina Governor's Institute
  on Alcohol, Inc.
Research Triangle Park, NC

Kenneth Warren, Ph.D.
Director, Office of Scientific
  Affairs
National Institute on Alcohol
  Abuse and Alcoholism
Rockville, MD

Barbara Webb, Ph.D.
Postdoctoral Fellow
Department of Neuroscience
University of Florida

Robert Weinreib, M.D.
Department of Psychiatry
Treatment Research Center
University of Pennsylvania

Constance Weisner, Ph.D.
Alcohol Research Group
University of California at
  Berkeley

Harry Wexler, Ph.D.
Center for Therapeutic Community
  Research
National Development and
  Research Institutes, Inc.
Laguna Beach, CA

Robert Zucher, M.D.
Director, Alcohol Research Center
University of Michigan

C

Plenary Lecture I

Avram Goldstein, M.D.
*Professor Emeritus of Pharmacology, Stanford University,
and Founder and Director, Addiction Research Foundation*

INTRODUCTION

My talk this morning will not deal directly with the main theme of the workshop—barriers to entry of young scientists into drug abuse research. Rather, it may contribute indirectly by presenting my overall view of the field, its problems, its accomplishments, and its opportunities.

This is billed as a plenary lecture. The dictionary definition of plenary, from the Latin, is "full"; but it doesn't say full of what! Full of enthusiasm, I hope, about the new possibilities in this *rewarding* field of research.

The workshop is about "strategies to raise the profile of substance abuse and alcoholism research." But what, pray tell, is a *substance*? And whatever a substance may be, the phrase "substance abuse *and* alcoholism," implies that alcohol is not a substance. These peculiar circumlocutions and euphemisms are political, not scientific, in origin.

Drugs, you see, are bad, and their use is illegal. Alcohol and nicotine are legal, so they can't be drugs. This peculiar distinction resulted in the establishment of two separate institutes, the National Institute on Drug Abuse and the National Institute on Alcoholism and Alcohol Abuse, the latter with its own constituency of alcoholics and recovered alcoholics—not, perish the thought, alcohol addicts and ex-addicts.

Rather than call drug abuse what it is, some well-meaning lexicographer thought to cover the whole field with a new term, "substance abuse," which

161

could embrace all the addictive drugs without offense to the standard hypocrisy. The problem here is not merely semantic; it reflects a profound gulf between the science and the perceptions of politicians and the public. One way we, as scientists, can raise the profile of drug abuse research among the politicians and public who fund our work is to educate them about the neurobiologic underpinnings of this curious medical, behavioral, societal disease.

I think an essential first step is to call a drug a drug. There are seven families of addictive *drugs*, which comprise the drug abuse problem. These are, in *descending* order of societal importance: alcohol, nicotine, cocaine and amphetamines, heroin and other opiates, hallucinogens, cannabis, and caffeine.

The field of drug abuse—substance abuse, whatever you call it—must seem a bewildering morass to the newcomer, especially to the young scientist trained in the cutting-edge techniques of molecular biology. Raising the profile of drug abuse research among scientists means identifying those critical questions that *can* be attacked by the most up-to-date techniques of molecular genetics and neurobiology as well as by carefully designed, controlled experiments on animal and human *behavior*.

Drug self-administration *is a behavior*—a remarkably specific behavior, for *just* these seven chemical families of drugs are self-administered, and laboratory animals self-administer the same drugs as do humans. All behaviors are determined in part by genetics, in part by environment. And all behaviors are rooted in neurobiology, in the anatomic structures and circuitries, and in the neurochemical processes of the brain. There was a time, not so many years ago, when animal and human behaviors could only be studied as *phenomena* in their own right. But molecular neurobiology has changed that dramatically, so that the behaviors we identify as drug addiction are beginning to be understood at the most basic level. Nevertheless, the fullest understanding of a behavioral disease will require multidisciplinary approaches, and the tendency of some molecular biologists to disdain less reductionist fields of research can be a hindrance to progress.

MULTIPLICITY OF DRUG EFFECTS

Any addictive drug has multiple effects, both psychopharmacologic and toxicologic, many of them unrelated to the addictive property. These comprise the ensemble of actions that make each drug unique, with its own special dangers for the user and for society. These special pharmacologic properties of each drug should be (but rarely are) taken into account in debates and decisions about our national drug policies.

The multiple effects of any psychoactive drug pose a unique difficulty in elucidating the neurochemical basis of addictive behavior. In studying other brain diseases, it is difficult enough to sort out which neurotransmitter or receptor abnormalities are causes and which are consequences of the disease. Any change in one brain system leads to consequent changes—some adaptive, some maladaptive—in other neural systems. The problem is compounded in the study of an *addictive drug*, for most of its effects on the brain will be completely unrelated to our main interest—the self-administration behavior itself.

For example, much research has focused on the prominent abstinence syndrome that results from stopping an opiate after prolonged chronic administration. Yet it turns out, as Aghajanian and his colleagues showed, that this is mediated at a different anatomic site (the locus coeruleus) from the mesolimbic pathway that mediates drug reinforcement. *Another example*: The disruptive effects of alcohol on psychomotor performance are certainly important for society—note this drug's causal involvement in half of all homicides and traffic fatalities—but they may have nothing to do with the addictive properties of alcohol. Multiple drug effects present major challenges to research design, for *anything* one chooses to measure in the brain after administration of an addictive drug is likely to be irrelevant to the addictive property of that drug. Such experiments have tended to measure whatever the current fad dictates—years ago it was biogenic amines, later it was neuropeptides, then NMDA receptors, then expression of early genes, now nitric oxide, and so on. Of course, we want to learn about *any* neurochemical change induced by an addictive drug. But what question about addiction does such a finding answer? And is the measured change a cause or a consequence of the addicted state? Subtractive cloning suggests an approach that is too little exploited—the search for differential neurochemical changes that occur only with self-administration but not with passive exposure to the same drug.

Research on the addictive process itself is a conceptual challenge. Addiction proceeds through three distinct phases, requiring study by different means, and offering different possibilities for intervention. We need to learn what neurobiology drives each phase: (1) the initiation of drug addiction, that is, the first self-administration and the pattern of subsequent use of the drug; (2) the full-blown active disease, that is, the compulsive persistence of self-administration; and (3) relapse, that is, the resumption of self-administration after a period of abstinence.

Phase 1: Initiation of Drug Use—Prevention Research

The initiation of drug use follows a typical pattern for all the addictive drugs. At the first exposure, usually in adolescence, some don't like the effects on cognitive function and mood, and they never become users. Some enjoy the drug and become (and remain) casual social users. Others like the drug at the outset, use it repeatedly, and eventually become compulsive, addicted, users.

These individual differences are present *before* first contact with the drug, therefore they *could* reflect innate genetic differences in predisposition. The best evidence for that comes from Cloninger's famous cross-adoption studies in the field of alcohol addiction. Also, abnormal responses to the drug, as demonstrated by Schuckit for sons of alcoholics, may provide a direct measure of vulnerability. In general, diagnosing special vulnerability at a young age could be a useful aid in targeting prevention efforts to those most at risk.

A fascinating recent epidemiologic study by Denise Kandel suggests, remarkably, that intrauterine exposure to nicotine during a woman's pregnancy predisposes her daughters to the use of tobacco in adolescence and thereafter. This result points to the need for more extensive animal research, in which prospective controlled experiments can be done (impossible on ethical grounds in humans) to examine the long-term effects (not merely toxicologic) of fetal exposure to each addictive drug.

For the study of genetic predisposition, reliable animal models have been developed— strains of mice and rats that prefer or avoid specific drugs in a free-choice self-administration paradigm. Thus, a basis for sorting out the relevant genes has been laid.

There is growing evidence that the "rewarding" properties of all the addictive drugs are mediated by dopamine release at the terminals of neurons originating in the ventral tegmental area and projecting to nucleus accumbens and basal forebrain structures. In one way or another—but how, exactly, is a current research topic—the various addictive drugs, acting through their own different receptors, impinge on this pathway. One would think it a simple matter to find or synthesize antagonists for the relevant receptors, and thus block the self-administration behavior. However, the "reward pathway" stimulated by addictive drugs plays an essential role in modulating normal, goal-directed behavior. Naltrexone, the specific opioid receptor antagonist, will indeed block the rewarding properties of heroin; but in practice, very few heroin addicts will use it. We do not really understand why; but naltrexone itself is mildly aversive to normal subjects, perhaps because functional opioid receptors are essential to normal mood and feelings of satisfaction.

A similar inference—that one must not perturb the dopaminergic pathway itself—can be drawn from the finding by Caron's group that knockout mice lacking the dopamine transporter (which *is* the cocaine receptor) are not affected by cocaine and presumably will not self-administer it; but they display grossly aberrant excitatory behavior, due to a persistent excess of synaptic dopamine. This elegant study ushers gene knockout technology into the drug abuse field. Of course, one first has to know which gene to knock out.

An interesting model analogizes an addictive drug to the vector of an infectious disease. Destroy the vector or inactivate it, and it becomes harmless. For scientists with a practical bent, here is opportunity to develop novel methods of prevention, treatment, and relapse prevention. One development, not yet commercialized, is a catalytic antibody to destroy cocaine more rapidly than the plasma esterases can. Another is active immunization against cocaine, reported by the Koob group in animal experiments. Neutralization approaches, based on binding and inactivating an addictive drug in the blood, have yet to prove their worth; stoichiometry, here, is likely to be a big problem, except for drugs used at very *low* dosage because of their high potency. A successful precedent is the commercially available antibody developed some years ago by Haber to counteract digoxin toxicity.

Phase 2: The Active Disease and Its Treatment

How best to treat the active disease is highly controversial—meaning, of course, that research has been inadequate. One school of thought holds that becoming drug-free is the only acceptable aim. Another holds that maintenance treatment, employing a long-acting surrogate of the addictive drug, can stabilize the addict's situation and permit social rehabilitation. If *research revealed a neurochemical deficit in the abstinent state*, whether antecedent to first drug use or consequent to chronic drug exposure, and persisting during abstinence, the maintenance approach to therapy would gain a more solid basis in neuroscience. Here the powerful new PET and functional MRI techniques might be useful. Thus far, although considered for several drug addictions, only opiate addiction is treated by maintenance.

Phase 3: Relapse and Its Prevention

What drives relapse after even long periods of abstinence? One view gives prominence to the abstinence syndrome, which is the immediate consequence of drug withdrawal. In rats, withdrawal is associated with decreased brain reward, that is, elevated thresholds for intracranial electrical self-stimulation. In humans, the feeling of "being sick," of "*needing* the drug," can drive drug-seeking behavior. But there is a problem. How do we account for relapse that occurs long after the abstinence syndrome has subsided?

Animal models date back to the pioneering work of Wikler, who first showed that conditioned cues play a key role. Current experiments by O'Brien's group demonstrate that drug-related stimuli can evoke craving and associated physiologic changes in abstinent heroin or cocaine addicts. A fascinating question is how a classic *psychologic* phenomenon—the conditioned cue—can activate the drug-seeking behavior. Whether this is mediated in the dopaminergic pathway itself or elsewhere in the brain is unknown.

Is relapse a consequence of irreversible neurochemical changes caused by prolonged chronic exposure to an addictive drug? Animal experiments show

that after a period of drug self-administration followed by a period of abstinence, resumption of self-administration occurs much more readily than in animals never exposed to the drug. This "priming effect" of the first small dose
after prolonged abstinence is thought to play an important part in provoking
full-blown relapse. Many research projects are suggested by the speculation that
the conditioned cue causes "priming" by release of an endogenous activator of
the reward pathway. But *which* endogenous compound? Acting *where*?

A recent study in rats by the Nestler group showed that an agonist selective
for Dl (but not D2) dopamine receptors can block both the self-administration of
cocaine and its priming effect after abstinence. An unexpected finding with
possible therapeutic potential, this work exemplifies the value of basic research
that is *consciously focused* on a drug abuse behavior.

It is noteworthy that millions of patients who receive an opiate chronically
in hospital are withdrawn and sent on their way without any desire to find and
use an opiate again. A difference between them and opiate addicts is, of course,
that they do not self-administer. But Lee Robins' follow-up of Americans who
became addicted to heroin in Vietnam did deal with classic self-administration
behavior; and yet very few of these veterans ever sought out heroin again after
their return home. This happy finding of a circumstance in which addicts did *not*
relapse adds an interesting fact to the relapse puzzle.

Quite interesting is the extensive evidence developed in China by Han concerning the neurochemical concomitants of electroacupuncture analgesia. In
animal experiments, he observed a frequency-dependent release of enkephalins
(at 2 Hz) and dynorphins (at 100 Hz) in spinal cord and other regions of the
central nervous system. Together with Terenius in Sweden, he found corre-
sponding changes in human cerebrospinal fluid after transdermal electrical
stimulation. Then it was claimed that the same procedure, in heroin addicts, re-
lieved the abstinence syndrome and inhibited craving. These provocative and
potentially useful findings have thus far been ignored; clearly, these data need to
be replicated and if confirmed, followed up vigorously.

Questions are raised by the surprising recent finding that naltrexone, a specific antagonist at mu opioid receptors, is beneficial in preventing relapse to
alcohol addiction. Does this imply that activation of an endogenous opioid system is what drives relapse to alcohol addiction? And would naltrexone be effective in preventing relapse in other addictions, too? Relapse, occurring even after
prolonged abstinence, is one of the key mysteries—perhaps the most important
one—in drug addiction research. We need to learn the circuitry and the neurochemical steps between the conditioned cue and the relapse behavior to be able
to intervene therapeutically. The truth is, whatever the addictive drug, clinicians
are able to bring addicts through withdrawal safely and comfortably. Thus, if we
could prevent relapse, we could make significant progress toward actually
eliminating drug addiction once and for all.

SUMMARY

If we understood the neurobiology of this strange behavior—drug abuse and drug addiction—if we understood the mechanisms whereby a drug *takes control* of a person's thoughts and actions, we might some day be able to intervene more effectively at one or another of the three phases. Especially useful would be techniques for preventing relapse.

There is a special challenge here for the young scientist who is not afraid to pioneer in a confusing area that needs innovative, creative ideas. There is a special appeal for those who would like to see their basic findings translated into therapeutic interventions with major societal impact on *the* most prevalent disease of our times. Finally, the field of drug abuse is especially ripe for interdisciplinary research, for the establishment of more centers of excellence in which molecular geneticists, neurobiologists, animal behavior experts, clinicians, and social scientists will collaborate *closely* (and *close* collaboration is the key to keeping a conscious focus on drug abuse) to increase our understanding of the peculiar compulsive and self-destructive behavior of the drug addict.

D

Plenary Lecture II

Ivan Diamond, M.D., Ph.D.
Professor and Vice-Chair, Department of Neurology,
University of California at San Francisco and
Director, Ernest Gallo Clinic and Research Center

Thank you very much for asking me to address the workshop. First, I will explain how I got started in alcohol research and afterward I will describe some of our more exciting observations.

Fourteen years ago, when the Gallo Center was organized, I had never done an experiment on alcohol in my life. I was a professor at UCSF when Mr. Gallo proposed that we build a center devoted to the neural basis of alcoholism and alcoholic brain disorders. I was asked to create a program that would be unique, that would use new strategies to investigate alcoholism, and that would not merely duplicate what was already going on in alcohol research. How does one start such a program? I surveyed the alcohol research community in the United States and learned that no one was exploiting the power of molecular and cellular neuroscience to investigate alcoholism. Therefore, I decided to develop a program designed to uncover fundamental molecular mechanisms of intoxication, tolerance, and dependence with the expectation that this information would lead to new therapies for alcohol addiction and alcoholic neurologic disorders.

I was not able to identify young investigators in alcohol research who had similar interests. Therefore, with the help of my colleague, Dr. Adrienne Gordon, we recruited faculty who did not have experience in alcohol research, but who recognized an exciting opportunity to use cellular and molecular biology to investigate alcoholism and its medical complications. In addition, because we were based in a clinical department, I wanted to be sure that our work would have relevance to clinical problems. Therefore, we brought together clinical and basic scientists to create a critical mass of investigators, just as Avram Goldstein described in his address this morning.

Our strategy was straightforward. First, we wanted to use simple, homogeneous cellular systems to identify the most important molecular mechanisms that mediate the response of neural cells to alcohol. Whenever we could, we would extend our findings to circulating blood cells taken from alcoholic subjects to confirm the relevance of our observations. Once we were able to measure important cellular and molecular events, I thought we would be in a much better position to apply this information to the brain with all its complexity and heterogeneity.

What about the problem of alcoholism in our society? Two-thirds of the adults over 14 years of age in the United States drink alcohol. If you calculate how much alcohol is produced in America and divide it by the number of people who drink, the quantity of alcohol consumed is roughly equivalent to 10 gallons of whisky per person per year. Now, this is clearly not the case for each American. Instead, about 10 percent of the drinking population, or perhaps 7 percent of the public, consume nearly 50 percent of the alcohol produced in this country. These are the alcoholics we encounter in hospitals and clinics; a conservative estimate is that about 25 percent of hospital beds in the United States are occupied by patients who have alcohol-related problems. In San Francisco, I estimate that as much as 75 percent of patients at San Francisco General Hospital have alcohol-related medical diagnoses. Medical complications involve the liver, heart, and just about every organ system in the body. When you add socioeconomic costs to the medical costs, the burden of alcoholism and alcohol abuse to American society is estimated to be more than $100 billion per year. Parenthetically, this enormous cost to society is much greater than the cost of other major medical problems, such as heart disease or stroke. Yet, the percentage of the National Institutes of Health's budget devoted to alcohol research is trivial when compared to the research budgets for other research areas.

What happens to people who drink excessively? Everyone is aware of the characteristic intoxicated behavior produced by alcohol. The degree of intoxication can be correlated with blood alcohol levels, because there is a very rapid equilibration between alcohol in the blood and in the brain. Therefore, blood alcohol levels accurately reflect brain alcohol concentrations. Alcohol is a sedating agent and, when blood levels reach 500 mg percent, naive individuals can become comatose and even die because of respiratory depression. This happens not because alcohol destroys neurons, but because alcohol depresses neuronal function in the respiratory center of the brain, so that breathing stops.

Yet, not everything is as simple as these correlations suggest. Many years ago, Mirsky found that blood levels can be misleading. Here, I reproduce some of his studies with volunteers given alcohol to drink. After volunteers were given a few drinks in about an hour, intoxication developed at blood levels approximating 170 mg percent. These subjects would be considered "drunk" by most conventional tests. And yet, if the same individuals were given more alcohol and examined 6 hours later, they were considered to be "sober" even though their blood levels were now much higher, approximating 300 mg percent. Since the blood alcohol level tells us the concentration of alcohol in the brain, this improvement in behavior cannot be due to less alcohol in the nervous system. Instead, something happened in the brain to accommodate and adapt to the presence of ethanol. This is a short-term or acute tolerance. We also encounter more striking long-term tolerance to alcohol in every emergency department across the country. Here I illustrate a study of patients who came to an emergency department for medical care. They were asked the question, "Have you had a drink in the last 6 hours?" If the answer was yes, blood alcohol levels were measured. The results show that the average was 270 mg percent, and a few people had blood ethanol levels greater than 500 mg percent, concentrations that can cause coma or death. What I didn't tell you is that all of these people were considered to be "sober" on crude physical examination. Clearly, these patients were chronic alcoholics with remarkable tolerance to the intoxicating effects of ethanol. If you are interested in the world's record for blood alcohol levels, it was measured at UCLA in a woman who walked into the emergency department after having discontinued drinking 3 days earlier. She had symptoms of withdrawal and her blood level was about 1,500 mg percent. Clearly, some alcoholics exhibit a remarkable ability to tolerate tremendous amounts of alcohol.

Alcoholics begin to experience symptoms and signs of alcohol withdrawal when more than 6 hours elapses after the last drink. That is why alcoholics tend to have a drink first thing in the morning. Alcohol suppresses these symptoms. Perhaps the craving for a drink during alcohol withdrawal is the same craving responsible for alcohol addiction. Alcohol withdrawal is characterized by hyperexcitability, and the most dangerous problem is alcohol withdrawal seizures; these occur in the first 24 to 48 hours. Later, of course, withdrawing alcoholics may develop delirium tremens, a well-known hyperexcitable syndrome with dramatic symptoms and signs.

We begin to wonder how we could approach such clinical phenomena at a cellular and molecular level. We thought it would be possible to identify cellular tolerance as a reduced response to repeated doses of ethanol, or cellular dependence by an abnormal cellular response during ethanol withdrawal that would be corrected by returning alcohol to the cells. We succeeded in both instances.

Robert Messing at the Gallo Center was interested in the molecular basis of hyperexcitability, particularly alcohol withdrawal seizures. He discovered that neural cells in culture adapt to ethanol by increasing the concentration and activity of voltage-dependent calcium channels. Ordinarily, ethanol inhibited calcium flux through these channels, but when ethanol was removed from the cells, the increased concentration of channels mediated a tremendous increase in calcium flux during alcohol withdrawal. This could contribute to neuronal hyperexcitability. The advantage of working with a cellular system is that it is possible to identify the molecular mechanisms that underlie these functional adaptations. For example, Bob Messing discovered that protein kinase C was required for ethanol to induce up-regulation of the voltage-dependent calcium channel.

Indeed, levels of two specific isozymes of protein kinase C, δ and ε, increased dramatically with chronic exposure to ethanol, and it seems likely that one of these isozymes, probably δ, is required to mediate the action of ethanol on calcium channel up-regulation. These results indicate that an ethanol-induced increase in gene expression for a particular protein kinase C isozyme may set the stage for the molecular events that lead to alcohol withdrawal seizures. Ongoing studies in several laboratories now suggest that calcium channel blockers can prevent alcohol withdrawal seizures in experimental animals and alcoholics. The point of this illustration is that it would have been very difficult to identify this specific molecular mechanism if whole brain or heterogeneous brain preparations were used initially. Now, however, it is possible to produce transgenic animals with overexpression or alteration of specific protein kinase C isozymes to confirm their roles in specific adaptive responses to ethanol. This work should suggest that it is not possible to explain neural responses to ethanol merely on the basis of membrane perturbation and fluidity changes. Instead, it seems that regulatory mechanisms affecting specific membrane proteins are very special targets for ethanol in the brain.

Another example of a regulatory system affected by alcohol was developed in collaboration with Adrienne Gordon over the past several years. We have been interested in cyclic AMP signal transduction. When a neurotransmitter reacts with its receptor, as in this cartoon, adenylyl cyclase is activated via a G protein, $G_{\alpha s}$. The result is an increased production of cyclic AMP which then stimulates protein kinase A activity. With long-term exposure to ethanol, however, neural cells adapt by reducing cyclic AMP signal transduction. This desensitization affects all receptors coupled positively to adenylyl cyclase. The advantage of working with cells in culture was that it allowed investigators to determine the molecular mechanism responsible for these changes. We found that long-term exposure to ethanol caused a selective reduction in gene expression for $G_{\alpha s}$, and thus decreased production of $G_{\alpha s}$ mRNA and protein. This accounts for heterologous desensitization of signal transduction. Interestingly, these changes at a cellular level mimic physical dependence. Receptor-stimulated cyclic AMP levels are abnormally low during alcohol withdrawal and can be restored to normal by adding ethanol back to the cells.

Identification of these short- and long-term neural responses to ethanol made it possible to discover the molecular mechanisms that regulate these events. This slide provides an overview of the pathway we have identified. Ethanol inhibits a specific adenosine transporter to block re-uptake of adenosine into neural cells. As a result, cells exposed to ethanol accumulate extracellular adenosine, which then reacts with adenosine receptors on the cell surface. In this case, adenosine A2 receptors positively coupled to adenylyl cyclase stimulate the production of cyclic AMP to activate protein kinase A. This results in a heterologous desensitization of cyclic AMP production associated with diminished protein kinase A activity at the cellular membrane. As a consequence of reduced phosphorylation, the adenosine transporter becomes tolerant to ethanol inhibition. In other words, two molecular mechanisms, one, a model of dependence and another, a model of tolerance, are linked during cellular adaptive responses to ethanol. And yet, each can be studied separately, as I will show later.

I have told you about studies in cells. What does this mean in the real world of alcoholism? We have discovered the same mechanisms at work in alcoholics. The same kinds of changes are demonstrable in lymphocytes from actively drinking alcoholics; there is desensitization of cyclic AMP signal transduction and tolerance of the adenosine transporter to ethanol inhibition. This is most striking in erythrocytes from alcoholics where there is virtually no ethanol inhibition of adenosine uptake. All of these studies illustrate that mechanisms discovered in model cell systems in the laboratory have direct relevance to pathogenetic mechanisms in human beings.

We have pursued cellular tolerance and dependence in studies too extensive to detail here. First, we tried to determine how the transporter, which mediates ethanol tolerance, is regulated during adaptation to ethanol. As this slide illustrates, without going into experimental detail, we have discovered that the sensitivity of the transporter to ethanol inhibition is controlled by the level of protein kinase A-mediated phosphorylation. In turn, this appears to be regulated by protein kinase C (PKC) via a protein phosphatase. A theme emerging from our work and other laboratories doing alcohol research is that the primary targets of ethanol involve regulatory mechanisms, such as protein kinases and protein phosphatases. As a result, we began to think about protein kinase A and how it might be regulated by exposure to ethanol.

Recall that protein kinase A exists as an inactive holoenzyme with regulatory and catalytic subunits. When cyclic AMP binds to the regulatory subunits, the catalytic subunits are dissociated and free to catalyze phosphorylation at different sites in the cell. We were curious how ethanol affected this regulatory mechanism. If we examine color photographs of confocal microscopic images of neural cells showing the catalytic subunit of protein kinase A before and after treatment with ethanol, we see that under normal conditions, most of the enzyme is localized to the Golgi apparatus in the neuron. Cellular localization here is confirmed by concomitant localization with other Golgi markers and there is no evidence of the catalytic subunit in the nucleus of the cell.

In contrast, however, exposure to ethanol produces a dramatic translocation of protein kinase A catalytic subunit to the nucleus. The effect of ethanol is related to concentration and time. High concentrations produce translocation in hours; low concentrations take 2 to 3 days. With this illustration, you can see virtually complete migration of the catalytic subunit of protein kinase A from the Golgi apparatus into the nucleus; the nucleus becomes literally filled with the catalytic subunit and the enzyme remains there as long as alcohol is present. It would be of interest, then, to determine the consequences of protein kinase A translocation. First, a reduction in cytoplasmic protein kinase A explains the reduction in phosphorylation at membrane sites observed during adaptation to ethanol. Second, nuclear localization of protein kinase A has great implications for changes in the regulation of gene expression. These kinds of changes may well underlie some of the chronic adaptive and sustained responses produced by ethanol in neurons and in the brain. It remains to be determined whether protein kinase translocation occurs in all neurons or is localized to specific neuronal populations in the brain, like the nucleus accumbens.

The long-term consequences of adaptive changes involve changes in gene expression, which probably underlie the development of complex abnormalities such as addiction and alcoholic neurologic disorders. Moreover, changes in gene expression may help to answer a puzzling question in alcohol research: How is it that short-term exposure to alcohol produces functional and metabolic changes whereas long-term exposure causes structural pathology and disease?

Because chronic exposure to ethanol produces changes in cellular and molecular function that require selective changes in gene expression, Michael Miles at the Gallo Center searched for evidence that specific kinds of genes are either "turned on" or turned off" by ethanol. He has already identified a family of ethanol-responsive genes. In this slide, it is clear that there is a selective increase in gene expression for some genes, including several stress protein genes. In order to study the regulation of ethanol-responsive genes, Dr. Miles coupled the promoter from an ethanol responsive gene to a reporter enzyme, chloramphenicol acetyltransferase (CAT). Now, assays of CAT activity can be used to identify factors that confer ethanol sensitivity. This will take us a long way in determining important regulatory mechanisms that mediate ethanol sensitivity and designing new therapies specifically to prevent or reverse adverse responses.

So, in a few short years, investigators at the Gallo Center have moved from behavioral concepts such as tolerance and dependence to selective effects of ethanol on gene expression and the regulation of signal transduction mechanisms in the cell. Undoubtedly, these changes contribute to altered complex behaviors, such as addiction, and the development of alcoholic brain disorders, such as dementia. This should not be surprising since CNS responses are ultimately regulated by the genes that control neural cell function.

As we accumulate increasing evidence of a role for gene expression in responding to ethanol, and perhaps conferring vulnerability to alcoholism, we can exploit advances in complex organisms in which behaviors can be linked to gene expression more easily than in human beings. Here is a slide highlighting some ethanol-induced behaviors in one such preparation. Acute exposure to ethanol first produces incoordination, then hyperactivity, and finally drowsiness and sleep. After awakening, there is transient incoordination, followed by a complete recovery. Although these behaviors resemble the effects of alcohol in human beings, this preparation is not a mammal, it is a fruitfly. Ulrike Heberlein has developed a *Drosophila* genetics laboratory at the Gallo Center to identify genes that mediate ethanol responses and perhaps to identify candidate genes that may be linked to genetic vulnerability for alcoholism in affected patients. We believe this new strategy will be of major importance in alcohol research because we know a great deal about the *Drosophila* genome, that genes controlling regulatory functions appear to be conserved throughout the animal kingdom, and that regulatory genes appear to be major targets for ethanol. Here, then, is a unique strategy: Exploit the validity of *Drosophila* as a model for learning, for behavior, and for responses to addictive agents. In the next few slides I want to show you how rapidly Ulrike Heberlein's work has progressed.

First, you need a way to measure ethanol sensitivity in fruitflies. For this, Dr. Heberlein uses something she calls an "inebriometer." The design is based on a model prepared by Howard Nash and Ken Weber to study anesthetic agents. You can see that the apparatus consists of a column about 4 feet, 6 inches long containing a series of incomplete soft platforms placed along the length of the column. The normal fly introduced into this column will remain at the top because of negative geotaxis. By contrast, a dead fly introduced into the top of the column would bounce down the platforms and come out at the bottom. So it is very easy to separate living flies from dead flies.

The column is prepared so that ethanol vapor can be introduced. Now flies become intoxicated, and, as they become increasingly uncoordinated, they fall to different levels in the column, holding on to different platforms as they fall down. When collected over time, the flies elute in a bell-shaped curve. This slide shows how the flies can then be separated by column chromatography according to their ethanol sensitivity. Populations of flies can be generated that are either very sensitive or resistant to ethanol intoxication.

One of the advantages of *Drosophila* is that it is possible to identify genes that control these kinds of behaviors. It is also possible to introduce random mutations into the genome and then screen for abnormal behaviors. If a behavior is identified, it is then possible to work back to the mutated gene. This approach is theoretically possible in animals, but is much more easily done with thousands of flies. Dr. Heberlein has introduced one mutation per chromosome and screened 50,000 flies. She has already identified more than a dozen mutants with increased or decreased sensitivity to ethanol and she should be identifying the responsible gene(s) in the next few months. Moreover, it is also possible to use available mutants as controls to prove that ethanol sensitivity is mediated by the nervous system and not due to an artifact. Perhaps this is best illustrated by the frequently asked question whether ethanol metabolism contributes to prolonged intoxication and increased sensitivity. Null mutants for alcohol dehydrogenase are available and when studied in the inebriometer, the elution profile is the same as wild-type flies. The only difference is that the eluted flies wake up slowly since they take a long time to clear ethanol because they are deficient in alcohol dehydrogenase. Clearly, sensitivity to ethanol in *Drosophila* cannot be explained by a failure to metabolize ethanol in the null mutants. In the slides to follow I show you examples of ethanol tolerance, ethanol sensitivity, and the fact that tolerance can be produced and studied for more than 20 hours after exposure to ethanol. Unusual tolerance to intoxication in flies may be particularly important, since Marc Schuckit has shown that resistance to intoxicating effects of alcohol may be linked to genetic alcoholism and the development of alcoholism 10 years later.

Think of the potential of this strategy: not only is it possible to identify genes that mediate normal and abnormal CNS responses to ethanol, it will be possible to test candidate genes in *Drosophila* derived from other systems to determine whether they contribute to ethanol-induced changes in neural function. In addition, genes identified in *Drosophila* can be used to identify genes in human beings. Perhaps those genes play a major role in mediating ethanol responses in alcoholics. Finally, genes that mediate and modify ethanol responses may be candidate genes for genetic alcoholism. The great advantage of *Drosophila* is that it is possible to move rapidly back and forth from complex behaviors to genes of importance. This is not easily done with mice, rats, or human beings.

E

History of Drug Addiction Research: Key Discoveries/Events, National Policies, and Funding

APPENDIX E History of Drug Addiction Research: Key Discoveries/Events, National Policies, and Funding

Event	Funding	Historical Time Line	Theme
Dr. Benjamin Rush, a signer of the Declaration of Independence and surgeon general of the Continental Army, was one of the pioneers of drug addiction research in the new America.		**1784** Pioneer researcher in substance abuse, Dr. Benjamin Rush, published a pamphlet entitled, "An Inquiry into the Effects of Ardent Spirits on the Mind and Body"	**Morphine and Pain Control**
		1806 F.W.A. Sertürner, a German pharmacist, extracted the first addictive ingredient, morphine, from crude opium, revolutionizing pain control	
Availability of morphine and the new hypodermic syringe during the Civil War created the "army disease."		**1868** Congress enacted the Pharmacy Act, requiring registration of individuals dispensing drugs	
		1875 Key elements of human addiction to morphine identified (e.g., fixation, withdrawal)	
The Bayer Company sold cocaine in pure form, as well as morphine and heroin, through pharmacies beginning in **1898**.		**1897** Gioffredi's study on possible immune system antibodies to morphine or other toxins	

The soft drink Coca-Cola contained cocaine until **1903**, when it was replaced with caffeine.

Narcotic Control

1906 U.S. Pure Food and Drug Act required that fraudulent claims be removed from patent medicines and that habit-forming ingredients be disclosed

1908 Nobel Prize winner Elie Metchnikoff's work helped to develop the theory of "autointoxication" related to narcotic dependence

1909 International Opium Commission convened in Shanghai to begin international discussions concerning the problems of narcotics and the narcotics trade

Congress banned opium imports

Substance Abuse and Criminality

1913 Rockefeller Institute created the Bureau of Social Hygiene to study drug addiction and its role in society and impact on criminality

1914 Valenti's study of the hypothesis that toxins produce abstinence effects

continues

APPENDIX E Continued

Event	Funding	Historical Time Line	Theme
Around World War I, a growing fear of drug addiction prompted more and more restrictive legislation to prevent easy access to drugs. The Harrison Anti-Narcotics Act of **1914** set forth a 6-year federal effort to control distribution of opiates and cocaine. In **1915**, doctors who prescribed narcotics to addicts to help them avoid withdrawal were prosecuted.		Congress passed the Harrison Anti-Narcotic Act, which began to regulate the production and sale of opiates and cocaine	
		1919 Supreme Court ratified the Harrison Anti-Narcotic Act in *Webb et al., v. United States*, holding that doctors may not prescribe maintenance supplies of narcotics to addicts	
		18th Amendment to prohibit alcohol is ratified	**Alcohol Prohibition**
		1920 The Rockefeller Institute's Bureau of Social Hygiene established a Committee on Drug Addiction to study and publish reports on addiction	
		E.J. Pellini, assistant city chemist of New York, rebutted Gioffredi's and Valenti's claims and stated that addiction and withdrawal had no organic basis and that those phenomena were "functional" or "psychological"	**Addiction Perceived as Psychological**

The Bureau of Social Hygiene gave $186,500 to the National Research Council (NRC) Committee on Drug Addiction	**1921** Narcotics Division established within the Prohibition Unit of the Treasury Department	
	1929 Bureau of Social Hygiene transferred its support of research to the NRC's standing Committee on Drug Addiction; the committee included medical school researchers and key governmental scientists and administrators, including the future head of the Federal Bureau of Narcotics, H.J. Anslinger	
	1930 President Hoover created the Federal Bureau of Narcotics, led by Harry Anslinger, precursor to the modern day drug czar, under the Treasury Department	
	1933 The 21st Amendment repealed Prohibition	**Prohibition Repealed**
$65,000 working budget for Lexington Narcotic Farm	**1935** First narcotic farm opened in Lexington, Kentucky, under the Porter Act for addicts in Federal prisons	
	Alcoholics Anonymous established	**Alcoholics Anonymous Established**

continues

APPENDIX E Continued

Event	Funding	Historical Time Line	Theme
	$663,330 overall budget for U.S. Division of Mental Hygiene, overseeing drug treatment	**1937** The U.S. Marihuana Tax Act (the federal government spelled marijuana with an "h" at this time) made the use and sale of marijuana without a tax stamp a federal offense	
	$103, 883 working fund for Lexington Narcotic Farm	**1938** Second narcotic farm opened in Fort Worth, Texas	
		1938 Development of a quantitative symptom scale for the severity of the opioid withdrawal syndrome in individuals by Himmelsbach and colleagues at the Addiction Research Center in Lexington, Kentucky (one of their first quantitative studies was of CNS drug effects in human studies)	
		1939 Meperidine (Demerol®) synthesized as first nonopioid narcotic analgesic (initially thought to be free of morphine's narcotic-like activity)	
		1943 Methadone treatments for pain were administered to soldiers in Germany during World War II when opium supplies were interrupted	
		1947 NRC established the Committee on Drug Addiction and Narcotics as the successor to the Committee on Drug Addiction	

continues

$12 million overall budget for mental health activities, including drug treatment, in Public Health Service

Alcoholism Defined as a Disease

1948 The drug disulfiram (Antabuse®) was introduced into therapeutics for treating alcoholism

1949 National Institute of Mental Health was established as the successor to the Public Health Service's Division of Mental Hygiene

1954 American Medical Association declares alcoholism a disease

1956 Congress enacted the Narcotic Control Act to increase penalties for the sale and possession of marijuana and heroin

1958 Synanon, begun in California, was the first therapeutic community

1958–1959 LSD was found to affect the brain's serotonin systems; stimulants were found to produce paranoid psychotic states

1961 Methadone maintenance developed from studies on a hospital ward in New York (Rockefeller University) by Drs. Vincent Dole and Marie Nyswander

APPENDIX E Continued

Event	Funding	Historical Time Line	Theme
		1963 The U.S. Community Mental Health Centers Act provided the first federal assistance to local treatment of addiction under the rubric of mental illness	
Psychedelics (LSD) appeared in the United States.		1964 U.S. Surgeon General declared that smoking cigarettes and other forms of tobacco was hazardous to health	
		1965 The term "drug dependence," meaning the psychological or physical dependence on a drug, arising in a person following administration of that drug or a periodic or continuous basis, is adopted by the World Health Organization (WHO)	**WHO Defined Drug Dependence**
		NRC Committee on Drug Addiction and Narcotics became the Committee on Problems of Drug Dependence; that name was changed later to College on Problems of Drug Dependence (CPDD)	
		1965–1975 Modern modalities of treatment for drug addiction began to emerge and develop	
	$504,000 for the Narcotic Addict Rehabilitation Act	1966 Congress passed the Narcotic Addict Rehabilitation Act for the treatment and reorientation of drug addicts	

$4 million for narcotic research for the Public Health Service's Mental Health Projects	**1970** U. S. Comprehensive Drug Abuse and Control Act consolidated drug laws and set penalties for trafficking according to each illegal drug's perceived harm	
	U.S. Comprehensive Alcohol Abuse and Alcoholism Prevention, Treatment, and Rehabilitation Act (Hughes Act) created the National Institute of Alcohol Abuse and Alcoholism (NIAAA)	**NIAAA Established**
	Congress passed the Drug Abuse Education Act	
Ford Foundation Drug Abuse Survey was initiated to estimate the prevalence of drug use in the United States.	Ford Foundation initiated the "Drug Abuse Survey Project" to pinpoint more precisely what should be done to combat drug abuse	
$6 million for narcotic addiction and drug abuse research allocated to the National Institute of Mental Health (NIMH)	**1971** President Richard M. Nixon declared "war on drugs"	**"War on Drugs" Declared**
	Establishment of the National Commission on Marijuana and Drug Abuse	

continues

APPENDIX E Continued

Event	Funding	Historical Time Line	Theme
	$6 million for alcoholism research at NIMH	1971–1978 Ford Foundation established the Drug Abuse Council to fund policy studies related to substance abuse	
		1972 President's National Commission on Marijuana and Drug Abuse recommended that laws against use of marijuana be relaxed	
		Congress passed the Drug Abuse Office and Treatment Act, which established the Special Action Office for Drug Abuse Prevention (SAODAP) in the Executive Office of the President. SAODAP lasted until 1975, when it was incorporated into the new Department of Health, Education, and Welfare	
War on Drugs began with the establishment of the Drug Enforcement Administration (DEA) in 1973 and the National Institute on Drug Abuse (NIDA) in 1974.		1973 DEA was established to control supply and enforce regulation of controlled substances	**DEA Established**
		Increased knowledge of the difficulty of maintaining smoking abstinence led to new views of relapse behavior	

NIDA Established	First demonstration (using tritium-labeled opiates) of the presence of receptors for morphine-like drugs in brain tissue by three groups working independently; this discovery initiated the extensive use of radioligand binding to study receptors for many types of drugs and endogenous transmitters in the brain and spinal cord
$22 million for drug abuse research to NIDA	1974 NIDA was established to give a national focus to the federal effort to increase knowledge of substance abuse; NIDA was supervised by the Alcohol, Drug Abuse and Mental Health Administration (ADAMHA)
	Congress enacted the Narcotic Addict Treatment Act, imposing federal control on the dispensing of methadone
$34 million for drug abuse research to NIMH	1975 Enkephalins discovered by Hughes and Kosterlitz
	1976 Demonstration of the opioid drug-like actions of beta-endorphin, a peptide found in brain, pituitary gland, and peripheral blood
	1977 CPDD becomes an independent organization
Nicotine Addiction	Schacter advocated a nicotine-addiction hypothesis based on studies demonstrating that when nicotine content was varied, heavy smokers adjusted their smoking rates to keep nicotine blood levels at a consistent level. He concluded that some internal control mechanism controlled smoking

continues

APPENDIX E Continued

Event	Funding	Historical Time Line	Theme
Rise in cocaine use occurred during the 1980s		**1978–1979** Development of the intracranial microdialysis technique led to direct studies on the dynamics of neurotransmitter release. This resulted in an increased understanding of the synaptic pharmacology of neurotransmitter systems and the neuropharmacological basis of normal and abnormal behavioral reactions	
		1978 Congress authorized law enforcement agencies to seize the assets of drug dealers, including money, real estate, and vehicles	
		Demonstration by Aghajanian of the important role of the locus coeruleus in the expression of withdrawal symptoms in opioid dependence	
		1979 Cloning by Japanese scientists of the genes for the three families of endogenous opioid peptides: pro-opiomelanocortin, proenkephalin, and prodynorphin	
A plane crash on the aircraft carrier USS Nimitz in **1981** led to drug testing of military personnel.		**1981** Demonstration that behavioral reinforcement (reward) induced by heroin is dependent on dopamine release in the brain	
		Congress passed a block grant program to give states more control over drug abuse treatment and prevention services	

$28 million for research to NIDA

1982 Sequencing of gene for the nicotinic cholinergic receptor at the neuromuscular junction provided molecular basis for first cloned receptor

Smoking literature described self-titration, or self-limiting action, as a process involving a threshold or satiation point of dose intake that functioned to maintain nicotine at consistent levels that regulate consumption rates

Virus for AIDS identified in **1984.**

1983 Measures taken to defer intravenous drug users from donating blood

1984 Crime Control Act increased federal mandatory minimum sentencing provisions for drug-related crime

Naltrexone (Trexan™) approved for treatment of heroin and narcotic addiction

Test for detecting HIV developed and licensed in **1985.**

Crack Cocaine Appeared in the United States

$1 million for NIDA training grants

1986 WHO established a three-step analgesic ladder to promote compassionate and rational use of opioid and other analgesics in treatment of cancer pain

Athletes Len Bias and Don Rodgers died from overdoses in **1986**, awakening the country to the lethal implications of crack cocaine.

continues

APPENDIX E Continued

Event	Funding	Historical Time Line	Theme
	$130 million for NIDA research	**1988** U.S. Anti-Drug Abuse Act mandated the creation of the Office of National Drug Control Policy (ONDCP) and stiffened penalties for drug possession	
		U.S. Surgeon General's report stated that cigarettes and other forms of tobacco are addicting	
		1989 Worldwide heroin production reached an all-time high	**Heroin Use Increased**
U.S. forces invaded Panama and capture Gen. Manuel Antonio Noriega in **1989**. He is sentenced and imprisoned for cocaine trafficking.		President George Bush appointed William J. Bennett as the first "drug czar" of the new Office of National Drug Control Policy	
		First Drug Court was established in Miami; also known as "Treatment Court," this was a criminal-justice-run program to treat addicted nonviolent offenders prior to trial	
	$194 million for NIDA research	**1990** NIDA's Medications Development Division was established to develop new medications for the treatment of drug addiction	
	$4 million for NIAAA training grants and $118 million for research	**1991** Supreme Court upheld a Michigan law imposing a mandatory life sentence without possibility of parole to anyone convicted of possessing more than 650 grams of cocaine	

$7 million for NIDA training grants and $230 million for research	1992 NIDA and NIAAA became part of the National Institutes of Health, U.S. Department of Health and Human Services (DHHS)
	1992–1993 Mu, kappa, and delta receptors in the brain were cloned and sequenced, leading to a greater understanding of the pathogenesis of opioid addiction
	1993 Supreme Court ruled that officials may not seize property acquired with the proceeds of illegal drug sales if the owner is unaware of the source of those funds
	Society of Americans in Recovery (SOAR), the first modern consumer advocacy group, was established; it disbanded 2 years later due to management problems and difficulty enlisting support from "recently" recovered individuals
	LAAM (Orlaam®) approved for treatment of narcotic addiction
	1994 DHHS adopted and published AHCPR/WHO guidelines for use of analgesics in cancer pain, including chronic high-dose use of opioids
	Naltrexone (ReVia™) approved for treatment of alcoholism

APPENDIX E Continued

Event	Funding	Historical Time Line	Theme
	$9 million for NIDA training grants and $331 million for research grants	**1995** FDA Commissioner David Kessler launched campaign to regulate nicotine use among adolescents	**Regulation of Nicotine**
	$5 million for NIAAA training grants and $142 million for research grants		
	$11 million for NIDA training grants	**1996** Nicotine chewing gum approved for over-the-counter sale; expanded public advertising of methods to reduce nicotine craving and dependence	

SOURCES:

Bureau of Justice. 1992. *A National Report: Drugs, Crime, and the Justice System.* Washington, DC: U.S. Government Printing Office.

Lowinson JH, Ruiz P, Millman RB, eds. 1992. *Substance Abuse: A Comprehensive Textbook.* Baltimore: Williams & Wilkins.

U.S. Department of Health and Human Services. 1994. *Preventing Tobacco Use Among Young People: A Report of the Surgeon General.* Washington, DC: U.S. Government Printing Office.

F

Recent Advances in Addiction Research

MOLECULAR BIOLOGY, BIOCHEMISTRY, BRAIN IMAGING, AND ANATOMY

General Issues

- Cloning and molecular studies on subtypes of key neurotransmitter and neuropeptide receptors, transporters, and enzymes involved in drug action.
- Dopamine systems: identification, cloning, and characterization of five distinct dopamine receptor subtypes; chromosomal mapping of human and mouse dopamine receptor genes; elucidation of mechanisms controlling dopamine receptor expression and signaling; cloning and characterization of the gene and complementary deoxyribonucleic acid sequence (cDNA) for the dopamine transporter; chromosomal mapping of human dopamine transporter; and increased understanding of molecular anatomy and regulatory mechanisms of dopaminergic systems in common reward mechanisms.
- Gene knockouts: evaluation of specific receptors, transporters, or enzymes in drug action by selective deletion from genome Transgenic animals: evaluation of specific receptors or enzymes in drug action by selective insertion into novel cells or animals and use of gene-selective switches to turn on and off transgene function.
- Signal transduction processes: role of G-proteins, nitric oxide, cyclic adenosine monophosphate (cAMP), phosphorylation, and other processes in drug action, tolerance, and dependence.

• Mechanisms of receptor sensitization and desensitization have been identified and are currently being related to mechanisms of addictive syndromes.
• Use of positron-emission tomography and single photon emission computed tomography imaging to evaluate drug action on dynamics of energy utilization and neurotransmitter function in living animals and humans.

Nicotine

• Characterization of the nicotinic-cholinergic receptor within the central nervous system.
• Demonstration that nicotine reward may be mediated by dopamine release.

Opioids

• Endogenous opioid receptors cloned and characterized (mu, kappa delta).
• Mu, kappa, delta receptor locations mapped in the brain.
• Regulation studies of opioid genes and processing of opioid peptides in normal and drug-treated states.
• Receptor cloning increases the likelihood of developing more selective agonist and antagonist drugs for each receptor subtype.
• Characterization of processes by which opioid receptor activation regulates neuronal function, secondary messenger systems, ion channel function, and gene expression.

Stimulants

• Specific interaction sites for cocaine and amphetamine identified on dopamine transporter.
• Genetically altered mice for dopamine receptors and transporter have produced exciting new models for role of dopamine in cocaine and amphetamine action and brain reward systems in general.
• Excitatory amino acids implicated in dopamine-mediated effects of cocaine; potential therapeutic implications.

Alcohol

- Identification of γ-isoform of $GABA_A$ receptor, which has high-affinity binding site for alcohol (i.e., alcohol receptor?).
- Physiologically relevant doses of alcohol (10–50 mM) shown to: enhance Cl^- flux mediated by the $GABA_A$-benzodiazepine receptor complex; inhibit Ca^{++} flux mediated by the NMDA-glutamate receptor system; and enhance Na^+ and K^+ flux mediated by the 5-HT_3 receptor.
- Acute alcohol effects on NMDA-glutamate receptor and downstream actions of increased intracellular Ca^{++} on nitric oxide production implicated in acute tolerance development.
- Chronic alcohol down-regulation of $GABA_A$-benzodiazepine receptor complex and up-regulation of NMDA-glutamate receptor complex implicated in chronic tolerance development.
- Low-to-moderate doses of alcohol increase the release of endogenous opioid peptides that may contribute to its effect on brain reward systems.
- Alcohol's effect on firing of dopamine neurons in the ventral tegmental area (VTA) and increases in extracellular dopamine in the nucleus accumbens (NAc) may also contribute to the positive reinforcing effects of alcohol.
- Serotonin, glutamate, opioid, and GABAergic neurons may modulate alcohol's reinforcing effects or mediate negative reinforcement from alcohol withdrawal.

ANIMAL MODELS, EXPERIMENTAL THERAPEUTICS, AND GENETICS

General Issues

- Expanded research into the neurobiological basis and behavioral mechanisms for "craving" and reinitiation of drug use.
- Use of animal self-administration models, place-preference testing, drug discrimination, and other behavioral models in conjunction with:

— in vitro and in vivo neurochemistry (microdialysis, neurotransmitter-selective electrodes, autoradiography),
— brain imaging,
— new strains of drug-responsive and nonresponsive animals,
— quantitative trait loci (QTL) gene mapping, and
— molecular biology (transgenic, gene knockout, antisense DNA).

• Mechanisms of somatic dependence established (locus coeruleus and other brainstem nuclei); predicted use of clonidine or other alpha-adrenergic drugs for treatment of somatic withdrawal.

Nicotine

• Development of a model wherein animals self-administer nicotine to blood levels approximating those of human cigarette smokers.
• Models for examination of "inhaled" nicotine.

Opioids

• Discovery of mechanisms by which opioids activate brain reward pathways (via VTA and NAc).
• Modulation of brain reward pathways by kappa agonists and antagonists; potential role of kappa agonists in blocking opioid reinforcement.
• Prevention and/or reversal of opioid tolerance and dependence by NMDA antagonists, CCK antagonists, delta receptor agonists, and nitric oxide synthase inhibitors.
• Substantial progress on molecular adaptations produced by acute or chronic opioids in the brain.

Stimulants

• Development of robust animal models of cocaine and amphetamine self-administration.
• Experimental evaluation of selective dopamine-subtype-selective agonists, antagonists, partial agonists, and other therapies as treatments for cocaine dependence.
• Demonstration that the neurochemical consequences of cocaine self-administration are different from involuntary injection of cocaine, suggesting different transmitter pathways involved in anticipation of reward versus behavioral response.

Alcohol

• Development of several genetically stable strains of high- or low-alcohol- preferring rats from common outbred animal stock.

• Experimental evaluation of opioid antagonists, serotonin reuptake inhibitors, 5-HT$_3$ antagonists, and dopamine D$_2$ receptor antagonists as treatments for alcohol dependence.

• QTL gene mapping of chromosomes associated with alcohol preference, sensitivity, tolerance, and withdrawal.

• Identification of genetic variants of principal enzymes of alcohol metabolism that influence alcohol drinking and dependence.

G

Recent Advances in Pharmacotherapy

GENERAL ISSUES

- Creation of National Institute on Drug Abuse Medications Development Division to evaluate new treatments for opioid and cocaine addiction in animals and humans.

NICOTINE

- Food and Drug Administration focuses on nicotine as an addictive drug; characterization of tobacco withdrawal syndrome.
- Demonstration that nicotine replacement is an effective treatment modality for a small but significant population of smokers.
- Nicotine chewing gum and transdermal nicotine patches approved for over-the-counter sale in 1996; nicotine nasal spray approved for prescription use in 1996; advances in other preparations.
- Increased research on nicotine replacement therapies for extending nicotine abstinence and reducing craving.
- Development of precise and practical measurements of nicotine metabolites, thus allowing better characterization of drug intake, dependence, and treatment outcome.
- Demonstration that addicted smokers regulate intake of nicotine to maintain specific levels in the body.

OPIOIDS

• Approval of LAAM (levomethadyl acetate, Orlaam®) as 2 to 3 times per week treatment for opioid dependence.

• Evaluation of long-term methadone or LAAM therapy in reducing illicit opioid drug use in many patients.

• Evaluation of buprenorphine and other partial agonist compounds as safer replacements for methadone treatment.

STIMULANTS

• Evaluation of catalytic antibodies for degrading or inactivating cocaine.

• Expanded evaluation of selective dopamine, serotonin, and opioid agonists and antagonists for cocaine addiction.

• Expanded examination of the concept of agonist replacement strategies and specific medications.

ALCOHOL

• Naltrexone (ReVia™) approved for treatment of alcoholism in the United States.

• Acamprosate (Aotal®) approved for treatment of alcoholism in Europe, and gamma-hydroxybutyrate approved for treatment of alcoholism in Italy.

• Expanded research into use of serotonin reuptake inhibitors, opioid antagonists, serotonin 5-HT$_3$ receptor antagonists, drug combinations, and other pharmacological treatments.

H

Recent Advances in Behavioral Sciences and Treatment

GENERAL ISSUES

- Demonstration of the effectiveness of psychosocial interventions in conjunction with methadone treatment for narcotic addiction and naltrexone treatment for alcoholism.
- Demonstration of efficacy of contingency voucher system as reinforcer for maintaining participation in drug treatment.
- Investigations of the substrates of cue-dependent craving and clinical approaches to minimize the likelihood of relapse.
- Identification of risk factors for using drugs (e.g., psychopathologies, personality disorders, difficulty in regulating emotions and behaviors).
- Identification of protective factors for prevention and treatment of drug abuse disorders (e.g., high school achievement, peer and family relations, participation in religious or social events, social networks, community reinforcement approaches).
- Identification of behavioral and social factors that serve as relapse determinants (e.g., psychological factors, drug availability and socializing with other abusers, emotional correlates and sequelae, craving, outcome expectancies).
- Evaluation of contingency management incentives that promote drug abstinence.
- Prevention strategies aimed at reducing the risk of needle sharing or unsafe sex to reduce risk of human immunodeficiency virus (HIV) transmission.

• Evaluation of joint pharmacological and behavioral strategies for cocaine and opioid dependence.

• Latent transition analysis (LTA) allows researchers to estimate and test models of stage-sequential development, such as the predictive effect of early caffeine use on subsequent drug use experience.

• Prevention strategies for adolescents and older youth have shown the value of delaying early initiation of drug use through school-based education and resistance-skills training and with increased availability of social networks, athletic programs, and neighborhood support activities for older children.

NICOTINE

• Characterization of the reinforcing aspects of nicotine in humans with appreciation of both positive reinforcers (e.g., cognitive effects, mood enhancement, weight control) and negative reinforcers (avoidance of nicotine withdrawal).

• Establishment of environmental tobacco smoke as a health hazard, with implications for air quality control in the workplace and public places.

• Successful patient-treatment matching studies (e.g., higher-dose nicotine replacement therapy for heavier smokers, supportive treatments for dysphoric smokers).

• Demonstration of differential etiology of smoking for men and women and gender differences in smoking cessation.

STIMULANTS

• Prenatal and other developmental exposure to cocaine may be influenced by both direct toxic effects and indirect effects of environment (e.g., parental functioning).

• Cocaine appears to increase the vulnerability of the exposed child to effects of a poor caretaking environment.

ALCOHOL

• Long-term follow-up study of behavioral effects of alcohol on young men with alcoholic fathers versus nonalcoholic fathers confirmed that a low-intensity response to alcohol at age 20 is associated with 4-times greater likelihood of future alcoholism.

• Twin studies show that vulnerability to alcoholism is determined by a combination of genetic and environmental factors.

- Mild cognitive impairments resulting from chronic alcohol abuse can affect an individual's ability to learn abstinence.
- Lowering allowable blood alcohol concentrations for young drivers reduces fatal crashes and arrests for driving while intoxicated.
- Training of alcohol servers in restaurants and bars reduces alcohol-related problems.
- Use of patient-treatment matching (Project MATCH) to establish new standards for alcoholism treatment research.

I

Key Barriers and Critical Strategies in the Research and Public Arenas

RESEARCH ARENA

Facilitating Integration and Collaboration

Barrier: Lack of Integrative and Collaborative Research Within and Across Institutions

Strategies:
• Develop collaborative agreements between deans, chairs, and administrators of institutions to participate in collaborative efforts and to identify individuals and areas for collaboration.
• Develop resource- and facility-sharing plans.
• Convene conferences, forums, and planning sessions to promote collaboration.
• Encourage multi-site clinical and preclinical trials and utilize direct funding to increase cost-effectiveness of research, clinical trials, and training at collaborating institutions.
• Develop mechanisms to involve industry (e.g., consortia, centers without walls, Requests for Applications [RFAs]).
• Expand forums and develop innovative mechanisms to present and share scientific information.
• Convene jointly sponsored workshops, seminars, symposia, and RFAs with different National Institutes of Health institutes.
• Integrate peer-review panels.

- Create "new" interdisciplinary centers of excellence.
- Create new funding mechanism for interdisciplinary research for young and senior investigators.
- Examine and possibly revise federal rules for research protocols (e.g., confidentiality).
- Educate Institutional Review Boards (IRBs) about the risks, benefits, and needs of addiction research.
- Encourage researchers to publish in clinical journals and other publications.

Increasing Skilled Human Resources and Improving Quality

Barrier: Lack of Educational Curricula

Strategies:
- Introduce addiction research at an early stage of education.
- Improve educational curricula in addiction research at all levels, especially among health professionals.
- Provide a progression of educational training opportunities and permit ready access to the study of addiction research issues.

Barrier: Lack of Certification Opportunities

Strategies:
- Clarify definition and requirements for expertise in addiction as it relates to specific specialties.
- Intensify training requirements and ensure that addiction is part of the educational credentialing process for all health care providers.
- Enhance educational curricula to convey understanding of concepts related to genetic, biological, and behavioral aspects of addiction.

Barrier: Inadequate Mentoring

Strategies:
- Enhance effectiveness of existing programs (e.g., K05, K07).
- Develop shorter grant review cycles.
- Ensure mentoring through innovative mechanisms (e.g., satellite programs or a network of mentors for co-mentoring).
- Implement a systematic assessment of the effects of mentoring experiences.
- Provide support for short-term internships in clinical settings.

- Develop joint programs with industry, foundations, universities, and government.

Funding Stability and Adequacy

Barrier: Low Levels and Instability of Funding

Strategies:
- Establish stable funding trajectory for research and training grants.
- Incrementally increase percentage of extramural research funding assigned to training support at National Institute on Drug Abuse and National Institute on Alcohol Abuse and Alcoholism.
- Develop joint programs with other agencies and institutions (e.g., industry, private foundations, academia) to support research training and ease the difficult transition periods for career development of researchers (utilize memorandum of understanding).
- Develop mechanisms to provide bridging support for promising young investigators (particularly at difficult transition periods).

Barrier: Attracting New Investigators

Strategies:
- Develop more effective targeting of specific awards.
- Encourage wider use of B/START (Behavioral Science Track Award for Rapid Transition) mechanism.
- Provide set-aside funds for summer internships.
- Provide travel money for conferences.

Barrier: Special Problems for M.D./Ph.D.s

Strategies:
- Provide a new fellowship that combines research and training.
- Provide mechanisms for longer training intervals.
- Develop a debt forgiveness program.
- Provide support for staggered or short-term clinical internships.

PUBLIC ARENA

Education and Training

Barrier: Lack of Education

Strategies:
• Launch a campaign to educate the public and others in the medical and scientific communities about the commonalities among addictive drugs.
• Emphasize the importance of addiction research and its accomplishments.
• Stress the complex nature of addiction—that it is a chronic, relapsing disease involving fundamental changes in brain circuitry.
• Encourage school- and community-based programs to address issues of addiction at age-appropriate levels.
• Promote the education of science writers through press conferences and public symposia.
• Encourage private and public funding of efforts to develop educational programs for schools, adult education programs, educational computer programs, or other media communications.
• Encourage the development of educational materials for undergraduate-level courses.
• Educate the public and professionals about myths versus scientific clinical facts regarding addiction.

Tackling Stigma and Building Advocacy

Barrier: Lack of Advocacy

Srtategies:
• Build advocacy groups from families of nicotine, alcohol, and illegal drug users.
• Emphasize what works and why and link research and treatment to other areas.
• Involve private foundations, industry, universities, and other organizations as well as M.D./Ph.D. scientist leaders to translate research findings and new clinical developments into lay terms.
• Increase communications with media to report timely, accurate, and reliable information about research findings.
• Disseminate scientific information to the public.
• Forge an alliance between local citizens' groups and scientists to conduct symposia.

- Organize grassroots organizations into a national network of advocates
- Aggressively seek increased support for research.
- Increase the visibility of addiction research within existing organizations that advocate on behalf of addiction treatment and services.

Index

A

Academic Career Award, 108
Academic Centers of Excellence, 6, 8, 135
Acamprosate, 81, 200
Access to substances, 62–63, 65–66
Accreditation and certification, 5, 106, 111
Acetylcholine, 40
Addiction
  behavioral effects, 45
  costs, 2, 11, 25–28
  definition, 1, 13–14
  multifactorial model, 13, 37–39, 48,
    162
  neurobiology of transition to, 42–46
  patterns of early substance use, 19–20
  risk factors, 47–49
Addiction Severity Index, 76
Adenosine metabolism, 172–173
Advertising bans, 58–60
Advocacy and consumer groups, 208–209
  competition among, 141–142
  for needs of addicted persons, 141–142
  recommendations for, 9, 146
  role of, 144–146
Age variation
  alcohol use, 22
  alcohol use, risk of, 47
  illicit drug use patterns, 20
  nicotine use, 22

rationale for early intervention, 19
substance use trends, 25
Agency for Health Care Policy and
  Research, 8, 134
Alcohol use/abuse
  access effects, 62
  advertising bans, 58–60
  age at onset, 47
  aversive reaction, 47
  costs, 2
  demographic patterns, 22–23
  detoxification, 74
  fetal alcohol syndrome, 58
  as gateway drug, 22
  genetic risk factors, 47–48, 174–176
  legal restrictions, 65–66
  media portrayals, 65
  neurochemistry, 40, 41, 45, 169, 171–
    176
  pharmacotherapy, 81
  prevalence, 21–22, 170
  price effects, 61
  psychosocial interventions, 79, 80
  recent research advances, 195, 196–
    197, 199, 202–203
  related morbidity/mortality, 22
  server role, 62
  social costs, 25, 27
  tolerance, 170–171
  treatment effectiveness, 73

211

treatment matching, 82
treatment settings, 75–78
use trends, 24, 25
warning labels, 57–58
withdrawal effects, 171–172
Alcoholics Anonymous, 76–77
American Association for the
    Advancement of Science, 97
Amphetamine neurobiology, 41
Animal studies, 39
    alcohol addiction risk, 47–48
    recent research, 195–197
    relapse processes, 165–166
    research needs, 164
Antabuse®, 79, 81
Antisocial personality, 57
Anxiety disorder, 57
Assessment and diagnosis
    addiction severity measures, 76
    in primary care settings, 63
    treatment setting decisions, 76
Attention deficit disorder, 57
Attitudes and beliefs
    moralistic view of addiction, 139–140
    as risk/protective factors, 3, 55–56

B

B/START, 7, 132
Behavioral sciences, 134, 201–203
Behavioral therapies, 79, 80
Board certification/examination, 5, 101,
    104, 106, 110
Brief therapy, 79
Buprenorphine, 85, 200

C

Calcium channel regulation, 171–172
Career development awards, 7, 116, 120,
    132
Career Teacher Training Program, 6, 108,
    109, 120
Causes of addiction
    conceptual model, 1, 9–10 n.1
    See also Initiation
Center for Substance Abuse Prevention, 30
Center for Substance Abuse Treatment, 30
Chemical dependency programs, 77

Clinical practice guidelines, 76, 79
Cocaine use/abuse
    crack/free base, 44–45
    demographic patterns, 19
    neurobiology of, 40, 41, 44–45, 49
    pharmacotherapy, 81–82, 164–165
    psychosocial interventions, 80
    treatment effectiveness, 73
    treatment matching, 82–83
    treatment settings, 75–78
Community reinforcement, 79
Conduct disorder, 57
Costs, 16
    disease comparison, 28, 30
    of drug abuse and addiction, 2, 11, 25–
        28, 30, 32
    health care, 2, 19
    indirect/related, 25
    morbidity/mortality, 27
    of treatment vs. interdiction, 32
    of undiagnosed addictive disorders, 63
Credentialing and licensing, recommen-
    dations for, 6, 106, 111
Criminal justice funding, 30, 33
Cues, behavioral, 46, 56, 165–166

D

D.A.R.E., 64
Delivery mechanisms, 44–45
    nicotine gums and patches, 86–87
Dependence
    definition, 13, 14
    neurobiology, 46
Depression, 57, 141–142
    in cocaine addiction, 83
Desipramine, 80
Detoxification, 74
    in opioid addiction treatment, 83
*Diagnostic and Statistical Manual of
    Mental Disorders-IV,* 15
Disease model, 1, 9–10 n.1, 13, 37–38
    pediatric onset, 19
    personal agency and, 48
    public education, 144
    vs. moralistic view of addiction, 139–
        140
Disulfiram, 79, 81

Dopaminergic system
adaptive emotional circuit, 43–44, 46
brain reward system, 39, 40–41, 164
drug effects, 40, 41
recent research advances, 193
significance of, in addiction processes,
2, 37, 49
Drug classification
by neurobiological effects, 45
opioids, 10 n.2
rationale, 15
stimulants, 10 n.2
typologies, 15, 162

E

Education and training in addiction studies,
16
funding for researchers, 121, 132–133
in medical schools, 5, 100–101, 103–
104
multidisciplinary approach, 104
obstacles to research careers, 95, 96–
97, 115, 133–134, 206
recommendations, 4–7, 97–98, 111,
132–133
role of mentors, 5–6, 106–109
secondary school level, 4, 97
for treatment professionals, 6, 109–111
Educational attainment, 21
alcohol use, 23
nicotine use, 24
Electroacupuncture analgesia, 166
Elementary schools, 4, 97
Emotional processes, in neurobiology of
addiction, 42–44, 46
Employment status, 21
Endorphins, 40
Environmental risk factors, 48, 56
Ethnicity
alcohol use, 22–23
nicotine use, 23, 25
prevalence patterns, 21
psychosocial risk factors, 56

F

Faculty
expertise in substance abuse studies,
100, 101

recruiting, for addiction research, 5,
106
Faculty for Undergraduate Neuroscience,
97
Families
advocacy role, 145
preventive interventions in, 65
risk factor for drug use, 56
Fellowship awards, 116, 120
Fetal exposure
to alcohol, 58
to nicotine, 164
research needs, 164
First Independent Research Support and
Transition, 120
Follow-up care, 74
Foundation awards, 131
Funding, 16
characteristics of individual awards,
116
for clinical investigators, 8, 133–134
federal, 30–33, 116, 118, 119–121
for interdisciplinary research, 8–9,
134–136
obstacles to research careers, 16, 115,
207
private sector, 32, 131
recommendations, 6, 7–9, 132–133,
134
system problems, 118
trends, 119–120, 121
vulnerable junctures in research
careers, 120–121

G

GABA, 40, 81, 195
Gamma-hydroxybutyric acid, 81, 200
Gender differences, 21
alcohol use, 23
nicotine use, 23–24
Gene knockout research, 164, 193
Genetic predisposition, 47–48, 164, 174–
176
Geographic variation, 21
alcohol use, 23
nicotine use, 24
Graduate education, 5, 111
opportunities for abuse studies, 99–100

Grant funding
    mechanisms, 116
    system problems, 121

H

Harvard Medical School, 101
Health consequences of addiction, 30
    costs, 2, 19
Health Research and Services Adminis-
    tration, 8, 134
Heroin detoxification, 74
High school, 19, 20

I

Illegal drugs
    alcohol use and, 22
    costs of addiction, 2, 11
    prevalence of use, 20–21
    social costs, 25, 27
    terminology, 161–162
    use trends, 24–25
Individual differences
    beliefs and attitudes, 3
    initiation of drug use, 162–163
Initiation
    age patterns, 19
    alcohol use risk factors, age-related, 47
    drug delivery systems, 45
    individual differences, 162–163
    peer influences, 56
    psychosocial factors, 2–3
    research issues, 55, 163–165
Insurance, 3
Interdiction, 32, 33

L

LAAM, 85, 200
Law enforcement, 32
Life Skills Training, 64

M

Media-based interventions, 65
Medical schools
    education and training in addiction
        studies, 5, 100–101, 103–104
    recommendations, 5, 106

Memory
    addiction process, 46
    neurobiology, 42
Mentors/mentoring
    recommendations for, 6, 109
    role of, 5–6, 106–107, 111
    strategies for enhancing, 108–109,
        206–207
Methadone, 83, 84, 200
    advocates for services, 141
    detoxification role, 74
Midwestern Project, 64
Minnesota model of alcoholism treatment,
    77
Morbidity, 11
Mortality, alcohol-related, 22
Motivation
    moralistic view of addiction, 140
    to use drugs, 45

N

Nalmefene, 49
Naloxone, 85
Naltrexone, 49, 81, 84, 164, 166, 200
National Alliance of Methadone
    Advocates, 141
National Cancer Institute, 118, 119
National Heart, Lung, and Blood Institute,
    118, 121
National Institue of Mental Health
    recommendations for, 7–8
    research funding, 118
National Institute on Alcohol Abuse and
    Alcoholism
    recommendations for, 6, 109, 132–133,
        136
    research funding, 116, 118, 119–120,
        121
    spending, 30
National Institute on Drug Abuse
    recommendations for, 6, 7–8, 109,
        132–133, 136
    research budget, 30, 116, 118, 119–
        120, 121
National Institutes of Health
    recommendations for, 8, 132, 134, 135
    research funding, 116, 119, 121

National Research Service Awards, 116,
120, 121
Neurobiology, 2, 16
of alcohol effects, 40, 41, 45, 169,
171–176
current conceptualization of addiction,
37–39, 49
drug delivery systems and, 44–45
drug effects, 41, 44–46, 49, 162–163
drug-induced changes, 45–46
emotional circuitry, 42–44
model of addiction, 48
public education, 144
recent research advances, 193–194,
195–196
of relapse, 165–166
research questions, 49–50
reward pathways, 39–41, 45–46, 164
second messenger system, 40
transition to addiction, 42–46
vulnerability to addiction, 47
New York City, 28
NIAAA. *See* National Institute on Alcohol
Abuse and Alcoholism
Nicotine use/abuse
access effects, 62–63, 66
advertising bans, 58–59
cessation programs, 85–86
demographic variation, 23–24
economic costs, 2
gums and patches, 86–87
intrauterine exposure, 164
legal restrictions, 65, 66
media portrayals, 65
neurobiology, 40, 41, 49
place-specific prohibitions, 60–61
prevalence, 23
price effects, 61–62
recent research advances, 194, 196,
199, 202
social costs, 25, 27
treatment effectiveness, 73
use trends, 24, 25
warning labels, 58
NIDA. *See* National Institute on Drug
Abuse
Norepinephrine, 40

North Carolina Governor's Institute on
Alcohol and Substance Abuse, Inc.,
104

O

Opioids
addiction and relapse research issues,
166
detoxification, 83
methadone treatment for addiction, 83,
84
neurobiology, 40, 41, 44, 45, 49
recent research advances, 194, 196,
199
substances classed as, 10 n.2, 15 n.3
treatment strategies, 83
Orlaam⁶⁰, 85, 200

P

Parkinson's disease, 2
Patient-treatment matching, 4, 82–83
Peer relations, 56
preventive interventions based on, 64
Personality trait risk factors, 56
Pharmacotherapy
cocaine use, 81–82, 164–165
education, substance abuse studies in,
100
opioid addiction, 83, 84–85
with psychosocial intervention, 80
recent research advances, 199–200
research challenges, 87
role of, 81
treatment matching, 82
Ph.D. programs, 133
recommendations for, 6, 109
Phoenix House, 78
Polysubstance abuse, 15
Posttraumatic stress disorder, 46
Pregnancy, 57–58, 164
Prevalence
age patterns, 20
alcohol use/abuse, 21–22, 170
ethnicity patterns, 21
trends, 20–21
of use by drug type, 15

Preventive interventions
advertising restrictions, 58–60
family-based, 65
federal funding, 30, 32–33
indicated, 3, 57
law-based, 65–66
media-based, 65
no-smoking areas, 60–61
peer-based, 64
price controls, 61–62
in primary care settings, 63
private spending, 32
psychosocial factors, 2–3
rationale for early intervention, 10–20,
163–164
restricting access for children, 62–63
in schools, 63–64
selective, 3, 57
target types, 3
universal, 3, 57
warning labels, 57–58
See also Relapse prevention
Primary care medicine, 63
education in substance abuse issues,
103–104, 110
nicotine cessation interventions, 85–86
recommendations for education and
training, 8, 134
Private sector
recommendations for, 7, 132
research careers in, 131
spending, 32
Professional societies
board certification/continuing
education in abuse specialties, 5,
110–111
recommendations for, 4–5, 98
Protective factors, 3
Protein kinases, 171–172, 173–174
Psychosocial functioning
alcohol server interactions, 62
co-occuring psychiatric disorders and
substance use, 56–57
effects of advertising, 58–60
initiation of drug use, 2–3
peer relations, 56
personality traits as risk factors, 56

psychiatric/psychological practice
specialization, 110
research challenges, 66
research issues, 55
treatment strategies, 79–80
Psychotropic drugs, 14
Public awareness and education, 16, 208
advertising bans, 58–60
advocacy for addiction services, 141–
142, 208–209
barriers to research, 142
content, 9
importance of, for research efforts, 9,
139
media-based interventions, 65
moralistic view of addiction, 139–140
recommendations for, 9, 144
school-based interventions, 63–64
selective preventive interventions, 3,
57
trends in substance use and, 24
universal preventive interventions, 3,
57
warning labels, 57–58

R

Rehabilitation, 74
Reimbursement issues, 3
Relapse prevention, 74
opioid addiction treatment, 84
psychosocial interventions, 80
research issues, 165–166
Research
career pathways, 96, 115
clinical, 8, 133–134
collaborative interdisciplinary, 8–9,
134–136, 167, 205–206
competition among researchers, 131–
132
federal funding, 30, 33, 116, 118, 119–
121
funding trends, 119–120, 121
historical development, 178–192
in initiation processes, 163–165
issues in addiction, 11–12
mentors, 5–6, 106–109, 206–207
obstacles to career development, 16,
95, 115, 133–134, 206, 207

opportunities in neurobiology, 49–50, 167

private sector, 131

psychosocial, challenges in, 66

public awareness/support, 9, 139, 142

rationale, 28–30

recent advances in behavioral sciences, 201–203

recent advances in neurochemistry, 193–197

recent advances in pharmacotherapy, 199–200

recommendations for education and training, 5–7, 106, 132–133

recommendations for funding, 6–9, 132, 133, 134

in relapse processes, 165–166

role models, 97, 107

shortcomings in education and training for, 95, 96–97, 206–207

social stigma as obstacle to, 140

treatment issues, 4, 87, 109–110, 165

vulnerable junctures in career development, 120–121

Risk of abuse/addiction

access, 62

current understanding, 47

environmental factors, 48

genetic predisposition, 47–48, 174–176

Robert Wood Johnson Foundation, 131

S

SAMHSA. *See* Substance Abuse and Mental Health Services Administration

Schools, public education campaigns in, 144

Secondary schools

addiction curricula, 97

recommendations for, 4, 97–98

Self-control training, 79

Self-esteem, 64

Self-medication, 56–57

Senior Scientist Award, 108

Serotonergic system, 40, 44

Smoking. *See* Nicotine use/abuse

Social skills training, 80

Stimulants

recent research advances, 194, 196, 199, 202

substances classed as, 10 n.2, 15 n.3

Stress and coping, 80

Substance Abuse and Mental Health Services Administration

programs, 30–32

purpose, 30

recommendations for, 8, 134

Support groups, 74

T

Therapeutic communities, 77–78

Tolerance

to alcohol effects, 170–171

definition, 13

neurobiology, 45–46

Treatment, 16

cue-dependent memory, 46, 56

detoxification, 74

effectiveness, 3–4, 32, 73–74, 79, 87

federal funding, 30, 32–33

follow-up, 74

historical development, 178–192

implications of model of addiction, 2, 48–49, 50, 75

length of, 76

nicotine cessation programs, 85–87

opioid addiction, 83–85

outcome determinants, 4, 74, 75

patient-treatment matching, 4, 82–83

pharmacotherapy, 80, 81–82

private spending, 32

psychosocial, 79–80

recent advances in behavioral sciences research, 201–203

recent advances in pharmacotherapy research, 199–200

recommendations for professional education and certification, 6, 109–111

rehabilitation stage, 74

relapse prevention, 74, 80

research issues, 4, 87, 109–110, 165

settings, 75–78

social stigma as obstacle to, 140

stages of, 74

support groups, 74
variation in services, 4, 74–75

U

Undergraduate education, 4–5, 98
University of Pennsylvania Medical
    School, 101
Use
    definition, 13 n.1
    neurobiology of transition to addiction,
    42–46

W

Warning labels, 57–58
White House Office of National Drug
    Control Policy, 9, 136
Withdrawal, 45
    alcohol, 171–172
    opioid, 83, 85
Workplace costs of substance abuse, 11
World Health Organization, 15